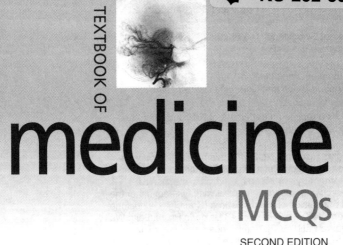

TEXTBOOK OF

medicine
MCQs

SECOND EDITION

Edited by

R.L. Souhami MD FRCP FRCR
Dean of the Faculty of Clinical Sciences,
Professor of Medicine,
University College London Medical School,
London, UK

J. Moxham MD FRCP
Dean of the Faculty of Clinical Medicine
Professor of Respiratory Medicine,
King's College School of Medicine and Dentistry;
Consultant Physician, King's College Hospital
London, UK

Andrew R. Freedman MA MD MRCP
Senior Lecturer in Infectious Diseases, University of Wales College of Medicine;
Consultant Physician, University Hospital of Wales, Cardiff, UK

Graham C. Toms MD FRCP
Consultant Physician and Endocrinologist, Havering Hospitals NHS Trust,
Romford, Essex, UK

Richard A. Watts MA DM MRCP
Consultant Rheumatologist, Ipswich Hospital NHS Trust, Ipswich, UK

Richard H. Evans MRCP
Lecturer in Medicine, University of Wales College of Medicine, Cardiff, UK

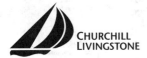
CHURCHILL
LIVINGSTONE

EDINBURGH LONDON NEW YORK PHILADELPHIA
SAN FRANCISCO SYDNEY TORONTO 1998

CHURCHILL LIVINGSTONE
A Division of Harcourt Brace and Company Limited

Churchill Livingstone, 1–3 Baxter's Place, Leith Walk,
Edinburgh EH1 3AF.

First edition 1992
Second edition 1998

ISBN 0443 06030 4

British Library of Cataloguing in Publication Data
A catalogue record for this book is available from the British
Library.

Library of Congress Cataloging in Publication Data
A catalog record for this book is available from the Library
of Congress.

Medical knowledge is constantly changing. As information
becomes available, changes in treatment, procedures,
equipment and the use of drugs become necessary. The
author and publisher have, as far as it is possible, taken care
to ensure that the information given in the text is accurate
and up-to-date. However, readers are strongly advised to
confirm that the information, especially with regard to drug
usage, complies with current legislation and standard of
practice.

The
publisher's
policy is to use
paper manufactured
from sustainable forests

Printed by Bell and Bain Ltd, Glasgow

TEXTBOOK OF

medicine

MCQs

For Churchill Livingstone:

Publisher: Laurence Hunter
Project Editor: Barbara Simmons
Copy Editor: Ruth Swan
Project Controller: Kay Hunston
Design Direction: Erik Bigland

Preface

This is the second edition of multiple choice questions in internal
medicine which has been prepared as a companion to the
Textbook of Medicine, 3rd edition, by four physicians who are keen
clinical teachers. The questions are designed for those taking
qualifying examinations and for MRCP. The MCQs book can stand on
its own but we anticipate that students will find it most instructive when
used in conjunction with the *Textbook.* With 1800 questions, across
the whole spectrum of medicine, the book aims to be comprehensive.
Each of the 300 stem questions has six branches and these have
been arranged, as best we can, such that questions E and F are more
challenging than questions A and B. The less difficult questions are for
undergraduate medical students in preparation for their qualifying
examinations and the more difficult ones for junior doctors preparing
for MRCP. In this way we hope that the MCQs book, in common with
the *Textbook,* will be of value to all young clinicians, during their years
at medical school and their early years of professional training.

London   R.L. Souhami
1998   J. Moxham

Contents

1. The epidemiological approach

1. **The following statements are correct:**
   A. A confounding factor is one associated with both the disease and the study factor.
   B. A systematic measurement error occurs as a result of chance association between the study factor and the disease.
   C. The incidence of a disease is the number of new cases occurring in a specified period of time in a defined population.
   D. The prevalence of a disease is the percentage increase in disease occurrence over a 10-year period.
   E. The standardised mortality ratio is equal to 100 × the expected number of deaths divided by the observed number of deaths.
   F. Life expectancy is equal to the standardised mortality ratio divided by the mean age of the population.

2. **The following statements are correct:**
   A. The relative risk of a disease is the prevalence of the disease amongst exposed persons divided by the prevalence amongst unexposed persons.
   B. The absolute excess risk of a disease is the incidence of the disease amongst exposed persons minus the incidence amongst unexposed persons.
   C. Prospective studies cannot directly estimate the relative risk of a given disease.
   D. Retrospective epidemiological studies do not require control subjects.
   E. Retrospective studies are unlikely to identify important causes of disease.
   F. The relative risk, of developing lung carcinoma amongst smokers is approximately 0.1.

(Answers overleaf)

1. **A. True.**
   B. False. These errors are a result of biased measurements.
   C. True.
   D. False. This equals the number of cases of a disorder present at a given point in time in a defined population.
   E. False. It is the observed number of deaths divided by the expected number of deaths × 100.
   F. False. It is defined as the total number of person-years of life lived by a group (of specified age) divided by the number in that group.

2. **A. False.** It is defined as the incidence amongst exposed persons divided by the incidence amongst unexposed persons.
   B. True.
   C. False. This is one of their main advantages.
   D. False. These studies are based on a comparison of disease cases with healthy controls.
   E. False. An example is the case-control study of Doll and Hill linking lung cancer with cigarette smoking.
   F. False. The relative risk is approximately 14.0 or greater.

3. **The following statements are true:**
   A. A single blind design prevents observer bias.
   B. A control group is not always necessary.
   C. Historical controls should be used if possible.
   D. An intention-to-treat analysis of outcome excludes non-compliers.
   E. An on-treatment analysis includes only patients who completed treatment.
   F. Treatment interactions can be examined by using trials with a factorial design.

4. **In screening tests:**
   A. The sensitivity of a test is the percentage of affected individuals with positive test results.
   B. The specificity of the test is equivalent to its false-negative rate.
   C. The odds of being affected, given a positive test result, is the ratio of the number of affected to unaffected individuals amongst those with a positive test result.
   D. The higher the prevalence of the disease the higher the odds of being affected, given a positive test result.
   E. The higher the prevalence of a disease the higher the specificity of the test.
   F. When using serum α-fetoprotein measurements in screening for spina bifida, the choice of cut-off level alters the sensitivity of the test.

(Answers overleaf)

3. **A.** **False.** It is the patient who does not know the treatment.
   B. **False.** Some form of control is necessary to judge the effect of the intervention.
   C. **False.** Randomised controls are best.
   D. **False.** The analysis is based on original treatment allocations alone.
   E. **True.**
   F. **True.**

4. **A.** **True.**
   B. **False.** It is equivalent to 100% minus the false-positive rate.
   C. **True.**
   D. **True.**
   E. **False.** Both specificity and sensitivity are independent of the prevalence of the disease.
   F. **True.** There is a trade off between high detection rates and high false-positive rates.

2. Clinical pharmacology

5. **The following statements are true in the study of pharmacodynamics:**
   A. Pharmacodynamics is the study of the action of drugs on the body.
   B. An agonist drug provokes a biological response by combining with a receptor. T
   C. The drug dissociation constant is the concentration at which half the maximum response of the agonist is observed.
   D. A competitive antagonist shifts the drug dose–response curve to the left.
   E. Non-competitive antagonists do not alter the maximum efficacy.
   F. α_1-Adrenergic agonists inhibit noradrenaline release at presynaptic receptors.

6. **The following statements are true in the study of pharmacokinetics:**
   A. The apparent volume of drug distribution is equal to the dose of drug administered intravenously divided by the concentration at time zero.
   B. Heparin has a very high volume of distribution.
   C. Drug clearance is not dependent on the volume of drug distribution.
   D. First order drug elimination occurs when the drug's plasma concentration declines in a linear manner.
   E. Phenytoin clearance falls with rising drug concentration.
   F. Bioavailability of a drug given intravenously is always 100%.

(Answers overleaf)   5

5.   **A.** **True.**
      B. **True.**
      C. **True.**
      D. **False.** It is shifted to the right.
      E. **False.** The maximum efficacy is reduced.
      F. **False.** α_1-Adrenergic agonists contract vascular smooth muscle.

6.   **A.** **True.**
      B. **False.** Heparin remains principally in the intravascular space and therefore has a low volume of distribution.
      C. **True.**
      D. **False.** The concentration falls in an exponential manner. Log transformation results in a linear fall.
      E. **True.** Phenytoin, salicylate and ethanol are examples of drugs that exhibit saturation kinetics as they undergo concentration-dependent metabolism.
      F. **True.** True by definition.

7. **The following statements are true in the study of pharmacokinetics:**
    A. At steady state the rate of elimination is equal to bioavailability.
    B. Propranolol has a significant first-pass metabolism.
    C. It takes approximately five half-lives of a drug to achieve a steady state.
    D. The half-life of a drug is dependent on the volume of distribution.
    E. Lipid-soluble drugs usually have a high volume of distribution.
    F. Weakly acidic drugs are poorly absorbed from the stomach.

8. **The following drugs can cause the following side-effects:**
    A. Oral contraceptives reduce the activity of warfarin.
    B. Ciprofloxacin increases theophylline concentrations.
    C. Cimetidine reduces phenytoin concentrations.
    D. Verapamil increases digoxin concentrations.
    E. Thiazide diuretics reduce lithium concentrations.
    F. Aspirin increases the toxicity of methotrexate.

(Answers overleaf)

7. **A.** **False.** At the steady state, the rate of administration is equal to the rate of elimination.
    B. **True.** By the liver.
    C. **True.**
    D. **True.**
    E. **True.**
    F. **False.** These drugs are mostly undissociated in the acidic stomach and are therefore well absorbed.

8. **A.** **True.**
    B. **True.** Fatalities have been reported.
    C. **False.** It increases phenytoin levels.
    D. **True.**
    E. **False.** They increase the levels.
    F. **True.**

3. Drug overdose and poisoning

9. In the clinical examination of the suspected overdose:

   A. The presence of focal neurological problems would support a diagnosis of opiate overdose.

   B. Pupillary dilation is consistent with tricyclic antidepressant overdose.

   C. Pupillary constriction is consistent with phenothiazine overdose.

   D. Hypertension is a feature of monoamine oxidase inhibitor overdose.

   E. Dystonia suggests overdose with beta-blockers.

   F. Hyperthermia is seen in salicylate overdose.

10. These specific measures may be valuable in these overdoses:

   A. Gastric lavage in a salicylate overdose taken more than 4 hours before admission.

   B. Activated charcoal and lithium.

   C. Forced acid diuresis with a severe digoxin overdose.

   D. Haemodialysis and ethylene glycol poisoning.

   E. Haemoperfusion and iron overdose.

   F. Oral cholestyramine and warfarin overdose.

11. In an overdose of psychotropic agents:

   A. Barbiturates account for the largest number of drug-related deaths.

   B. Forced alkaline diuresis is the treatment of choice in severe barbiturate overdose.

   C. Flumazenil will specifically reverse tricyclic antidepressant overdose.

   D. A wide QRS complex suggests a tricyclic antidepressant overdose.

   E. Gastric lavage is contraindicated in tricyclic overdose.

   F. Hypernatraemia may occur in lithium overdose.

(Answers overleaf)

9. A. **False.** Focal neurological findings are rare in metabolic coma.
   B. **True.**
   C. **False.** The anticholinergic action produces large pupils.
   D. **True.**
   E. **False.** This occurs with antidopaminergic drugs, e.g. metoclopramide.
   F. **True.**

10. A. **True.** Salicylates delay gastric emptying.
    B. **False.**
    C. **False.**
    D. **True.**
    E. **False.** The iron chelater desferrioxamine should be used.
    F. **True.**

11. A. **True.**
    B. **False.** Charcoal haemoperfusion is a much more efficient method of eliminating the drug.
    C. **False.** This is a specific benzodiazepine antagonist.
    D. **True.**
    E. **False.** This may be effective up to 4 hours after the overdose.
    F. **True.** This is due to nephrogenic diabetes insipidus.

12. In salicylate poisoning:

   A. A lactic acidosis may occur. T
   B. A respiratory alkalosis may occur. T
   C. Hypoglycaemia may occur. T
   D. Coma occurs early in overdose. F
   E. Activated charcoal does not prevent drug absorption following gastric lavage. C
   F. Pulmonary oedema may occur despite a normal pulmonary capillary wedge pressure. T

13. In paracetamol poisoning:

   A. Patients who have taken fewer than 30 (500 mg) tablets rarely sustain severe liver damage. T
   B. Renal failure can occur in the absence of liver failure. T
   C. N-acetylcysteine is effective only if given within 8 hours of ingestion. F
   D. Early hypoglycaemia indicates severe liver damage. T
   E. A prothrombin ratio of greater than 3 at 48 hours indicates severe liver damage.
   F. Excessive production of glutathione causes hepatic damage. F

14. The following are features of poisoning with these cardiorespiratory agents:

   A. Hypokalaemia occurs in severe digoxin overdose.
   B. Digoxin-specific antibody fragments are effective in severe digoxin overdose.
   C. Beta-blockers may precipitate severe asthma. T
   D. Clonidine can cause severe hypertension.
   E. Severe hyperkalaemia can occur in theophylline toxicity.
   F. Haemoperfusion is ineffective in severe theophylline poisoning.

15. The following symptoms are associated with poisoning with the following agents:

   A. Phenytoin and horizontal nystagmus.
   B. Quinine and blindness.
   C. Benzene and aplastic anaemia.
   D. Ethanol and severe hypoglycaemia.
   E. Methanol and metabolic alkalosis.
   F. Organophosphate insecticides and muscle fasciculation.

(Answers overleaf)

12. **A.** **True.** Salicylates interfere with normal carbohydrate metabolism.
    B. **True.** Due to stimulation of the respiratory centre.
    C. **True.**
    D. **False.** Coma only occurs late in severe poisoning.
    E. **False.** This may be effective.
    F. **True.** Mechanical ventilation and positive end expiratory pressure may be needed.

13. **A.** **False.** As few as 24 × 500 mg tablets can cause severe liver damage.
    B. **True.**
    C. **False.** This may be effective up to 24 hours after ingestion and even beyond this time.
    D. **True.** The commonest cause of early coma in severe poisoning.
    E. **True.**
    F. **False.** Glutathione normally conjugates the toxic paracetamol metabolites. Glutathione is depleted in paracetamol poisoning.

14. **A.** **False.** Hyperkalaemia occurs.
    B. **True.**
    C. **True.**
    D. **True.** Due to partial α-agonist activity. However, hypotension is more common.
    E. **False.** Hypokalaemia can occur.
    F. **False.** This is the most effective method of removal.

15. **A.** **True.** It causes cerebellar signs.
    B. **True.** It causes retinal oedema and optic atrophy.
    C. **True.**
    D. **True.** Particularly in children.
    E. **False.** It causes metabolic acidosis.
    F. **True.**

4. Physical and environmental causes of disease

16. **The following are features of hyperthermia:**
    A. Hyponatraemia is common in patients suffering from heat cramps.
    B. Peripheral hypothermia can occur in heatstroke.
    C. Beta-blockers are used in the treatment of heatstroke.
    D. Hyperglycaemia indicates severe heatstroke.
    E. Hypophosphataemia occurs in severe heatstroke.
    F. Renal failure does not occur if circulatory collapse is prevented by volume replacement.

17. **The following are true in hypothermia:**
    A. The core temperature is less than 35°C.
    B. The condition can be precipitated by phenothiazines.
    C. Shivering may be absent below 30°C.
    D. J waves may be seen on the ECG.
    E. The condition is associated with hyperpituitarism.
    F. Serum amylase levels may be elevated.

18. **In exposure to radiation:**
    A. The gray scale measures the amount of energy exposure that has occurred.
    B. Most background radiation is from radon.
    C. Bone marrow failure usually occurs within 5 days of exposure.
    D. The lung parenchyma is resistant to radiation.
    E. Intestinal symptoms occur only late in the course of severe exposure.
    F. With modern supportive treatment most patients will survive exposures of up to 10 Gy.

(Answers overleaf)

16. **A. True.**   Probably a result of hypotonic fluid replacement.
    B. True.   The core temperature must always be taken as peripheral vasoconstriction can lead to cool peripheries.
    C. False.   They may cause heatstroke by preventing circulatory adaptation to heat.
    D. False.   Hypoglycaemia indicates severe heatstroke and liver damage.
    E. False.   Hyperphosphataemia occurs due to muscle damage.
    F. False.   Despite rehydration, rhabdomyolysis can occur—leading rapidly to renal failure.

17. **A. True.**
    B. True.
    C. True.
    D. True.
    E. False.   It is associated with hypopituitarism.
    F. True.

18. **A. False.**   The gray measures the amount of energy deposited in the tissues.
    B. True.
    C. False.   Failure in 7–10 days is usual.
    D. False.   Radiation pneumonitis and fibrosis are common.
    E. False.   Above 15 Gy severe diarrhoea may be the first symptom to occur.
    F. True.

19. The following statements are true in exposure to extremes of barometric pressure:

A. Commercial aircraft cabin pressures are maintained at a pressure equivalent to 1000 metres.

B. A principal symptom of acute mountain sickness is headache.

C. A normochromic, normocytic anaemia often develops in chronic mountain sickness.

D. Decompression sickness is caused by helium from the inspired gas mixture coming out of solution.

E. Acetazolamide is ineffective in the prevention of acute mountain sickness.

F. A scuba diver can avoid a pneumothorax by holding his breath during a rapid ascent.

(Answers overleaf)

19. A. False. The pressure is equivalent to 2500 metres.
    B. True. It is due to raised intracranial pressure.
    C. False. Polycythaemia is almost invariable.
    D. False. It is the nitrogen which comes out of solution.
    E. False. It probably acts by partially reversing the respiratory alkalosis.
    F. False. If a diver breathes air below the surface he must allow time for the pressurised air to be exhaled, or the lung may rupture.

5. The genetic basis of disease

20. **In an X-linked recessive condition:**
   A. Half the daughters of carrier females are affected.
   B. Males hemizygous for the abnormal allele are affected.
   C. All the sons of a carrier female are affected.
   D. All the daughters of an affected male are carriers.
   E. All the sons of an affected male are carriers.
   F. Females heterozygous for the abnormal allele are affected.

21. **The following are true:**
   A. If two alleles at a locus are identical, the individual is said to be heterozygous.
   B. Chromosomes may be visualised by light microscopy.
   C. Restriction enzymes cut double stranded DNA randomly.
   D. The polymerase chain reaction is a method of directly amplifying specific sequences of RNA.
   E. Reverse transcriptase enables synthesis of DNA from RNA.
   F. Exons are coding regions of DNA.

22. **The following are true regarding chromosome abnormalities:**
   A. Down's syndrome is usually due to trisomy 21.
   B. The risk of Down's syndrome increases with paternal age.
   C. 47, XXX females are physically normal.
   D. Turner's syndrome individuals are phenotypically male.
   E. Klinefelter's syndrome individuals are phenotypically female.
   F. Down's syndrome may usually be diagnosed at birth.

23. **The following are true statements:**
   A. Anticipation is the phenomenon in which severity of disease increases in successive generations.
   B. Huntington's chorea shows expansion of trinucleotide repeats.
   C. Homocystinuria is an autosomal dominant disorder.
   D. Phenylketonuria is inherited in an autosomal recessive manner.
   E. The Guthrie test is used to screen neonates for hypothyroidism.
   F. Phenylketonuria is treated with a high phenylalanine diet.

(Answers overleaf)

20. A. **False.**   Half the daughters are carriers.
     B. **True.**
     C. **False.**   Half are affected.
     D. **True.**
     E. **False.**   Only the daughters of an affected male are carriers.
     F. **False.**

21. A. **False.**   Homozygous.
     B. **True.**
     C. **False.**   Restriction enzymes cut DNA at specific nucleotide sequences.
     D. **False.**   The polymerase chain reaction is a method of amplifying DNA.
     E. **True.**
     F. **True.**   Introns are non-coding sequences of DNA.

22. A. **True.**   In 95% of cases.
     B. **False.**   Increasing maternal age is associated with an increased risk of Down's syndrome.
     C. **True.**
     D. **False.**   They are phenotypically female with 45,X chromosome complement.
     E. **False.**   They are male, but have eunuchoid appearance with female fat distribution and gynaecomastia. The testes are small.
     F. **True.**   The appearance is typical.

23. A. **True.**   The clearest example is myotonic dystrophy.
     B. **True.**   Expansion of CAG repeat in the gene on chromosome 4p16.
     C. **False.**   Homocystinuria is inherited in an autosomal recessive manner.
     D. **True.**
     E. **False.**   The Guthrie test is used to screen for phenylketonuria.
     F. **False.**   Phenylketonuria is treated with a low phenylalanine diet.

6. Infection, immunodeficiency and inflammation

24. The immune response:
  A. B lymphocytes can present antigen.
  B. CD8 + T cells are helper cells.
  C. The T cell receptor is a member of the immunoglobulin supergene family.
  D. CD4+ T cells require antigen to be presented by HLA class II molecules.
  E. The T_H1 pattern of cytokine secretion favours an antibody response.
  F. Interleukin 2 (IL-2) secretion is a result of T cell activation.

25. IgG:
  A. Is present in normal human serum at a higher concentration than IgM.
  B. Has four subclasses.
  C. Has a pentameric structure.
  D. Has a molecular weight of 150–170 kD.
  E. May activate complement.
  F. Causes mast cell degranulation.

26. The following statements about hypersensitivity are true:
  A. Type II is mediated by mast cells.
  B. Immune complex formation results in activation of complement.
  C. Histamine decreases vascular permeability.
  D. Transfusion reactions involve a type II reaction.
  E. C3a causes mast cell degranulation.
  F. Anaphylactic reactions typically occur several hours after antigen exposure.

(Answers overleaf)

19

24. **A.** **True.** Dendritic cells of spleen and lymph nodes and Langerhans cells can also present antigen.
B. **False.** CD4+ T cells are helper cells.
C. **True.** Immunoglobulin and HLA molecules are other members.
D. **True.**
E. **False.** T_H1 favours a cellular response.
F. **True.**

25. **A.** **True.**
B. **True.** Each IgG subclass has a slightly different function.
C. **False.** IgG is monomeric, IgM is pentameric.
D. **True.**
E. **True.**
F. **False.** IgE causes mast cell degranulation.

26. **A.** **False.** Type I hypersensitivity is mediated by mast cells.
B. **True.** Via classical pathway.
C. **False.** Histamine increases vascular permeability.
D. **True.**
E. **True.**
F. **False.** They occur within minutes of exposure.

27. **The following statements about the HLA system are true:**

   A. The genes encoding the HLA system are in man located on chromosome 14.
   B. β_2-microglobulin is a component of class II HLA molecules.
   C. HLA molecules are expressed co-dominantly.
   D. Class II HLA molecules are expressed on all nucleated cells.
   E. HLA B8-DR3 is associated with autoimmune disease.
   F. HLA class II is composed of the A, B and C loci.

(Answers overleaf)

27. A. False.   HLA is located on chromosome 6; the heavy chain of immunoglobulin is located on chromosome 14.

B. False. β_2-microglobulin is a component of class I molecules.

C. True.

D. False.   Class I is expressed by all nucleated cells; class II by B cells, antigen presenting cells and activated T cells.

E. True.

F. False.   The D loci are class II; the A, B and C loci are class I.

7. Nutrition in clinical medicine

28. The following are true of dietary protein and energy requirements:

A. The energy requirement of an individual depends primarily on his or her level of physical activity.

B. Most of the dietary energy is required for pumping ions across cell membranes.

C. Energy requirement per unit body weight is highest in young adults.

D. Fats provide twice as much energy per unit weight compared with protein or carbohydrate.

E. Dietary energy is stored less efficiently during pregnancy.

F. Dietary energy requirements decrease with systemic infections.

29. The following vitamin deficiencies and clinical features are correctly matched:

A. Thiamine deficiency and ophthalmoplegia.

B. Pyridoxine deficiency and cerebellar ataxia.

C. Vitamin K deficiency and prolonged prothrombin time.

D. Vitamin C deficiency and glossitis.

E. Niacin deficiency (pellagra) and peripheral neuropathy.

F. Vitamin A deficiency and corneal ulceration.

30. The following are recognised complications of parenteral feeding via a central venous cannula:

A. Disturbed liver function.

B. Hyperglycaemia.

C. Metabolic acidosis.

D. Hypoglycaemia.

E. Hypercapnia.

F. Cardiac arrhythmias.

(Answers overleaf)

28. A. **False.** It depends primarily on body size and composition. Age, physical activity, environmental temperature and physiological state are also important.
    B. **True.**
    C. **False.** It is highest in infants and young children.
    D. **True.** A reduction in the fat content of the diet is a relatively efficient way to lose weight.
    E. **False.** There is a marked *increase* in efficiency of metabolism during pregnancy such that dietary energy is stored more easily. Many women in the UK date their obesity from the time of their pregnancy.
    F. **False.** Dietary energy requirements are *increased*. As nutrient intake is often decreased, there is a risk of protein–energy malnutrition in protracted systemic infections.

29. A. **True.**
    B. **False.** Cerebellar ataxia is a feature of thiamine deficiency.
    C. **True.** Reduced hepatic synthesis of vitamin K-dependent clotting factors.
    D. **False.** Bleeding gums is a feature.
    E. **False.** Peripheral neuropathy is found in deficiencies of thiamine or pyridoxine.
    F. **True.** A late and irreversible complication.

30. A. **True.** However, this is rarely an important clinical problem.
    B. **True.** A common occurrence, requiring insulin treatment.
    C. **True.** Can result from administration of fructose and excessive amino acids.
    D. **True.**
    E. **True.** Patients vulnerable to respiratory failure should not receive large glucose loads because of their impaired ability to excrete the extra CO_2 produced.
    F. **True.** A complication of (i) central venous cannula insertion and (ii) hypophosphataemia.

31. The following nutritional factors contribute to the aetiology of the stated disease:

A. Obesity and colonic cancer.

B. High dietary polyunsaturated fats and coronary artery disease.

C. High sodium intake and hypertension.

D. High-fibre diet and gallstones.

E. Aflatoxins and primary liver cell cancer.

F. Vitamin C supplementation and oxalate urinary calculi.

(Answers overleaf)

31. **A.** **True.**
   B. **False.** High dietary intake of *saturated* fats leads to raised serum cholesterol and VLDL which contribute to atheroma.
   C. **True.**
   D. **False.** Gallstones may be associated with a *low*-fibre diet.
   E. **True.**
   F. **True.**

8. Cancer medicine

32. In hormone therapy in cancer:

A. Stilboestrol reduces growth of prostatic carcinoma.
B. Steroid hormones are transported to the cell nucleus.
C. The presence of the oestrogen receptor is associated with an increased response to hormone therapy in breast cancer.
D. Tamoxifen is a progesterone analogue.
E. Aminoglutethimide is an aromatase inhibitor.
F. LHRH agonists cause a fall in plasma testosterone.

33. Complications of chemotherapy include:

A. Cardiomyopathy with anthracycline therapy.
B. Peripheral neuropathy with azathioprine therapy.
C. Pulmonary fibrosis with busulphan therapy.
D. High frequency deafness with cisplatin therapy.
E. A white count nadir 1–2 days after high dose intravenous therapy.
F. Increased risk of acute myelomonocytic leukaemia.

34. The following are true about tumour markers:

A. The acid phosphatase is elevated in pancreatic cancer.
B. Carcinoembryonic antigen (CEA) is raised in inflammatory bowel disease.
C. Moderate elevation of serum α-fetoprotein occurs in early pregnancy and in hepatitis.
D. Human chorionic gonadotrophin (β-hCG) is elevated in choriocarcinoma.
E. Measurement of carcinoembryonic antigen (CEA) is a useful screening test for colorectal carcinoma.
F. Human chorionic gonadotrophin (β-hCG) level is a useful predictor of relapse in testicular cancer.

(Answers overleaf)

32. A. **True.**
     B. **True.** In association with a receptor.
     C. **True.**
     D. **False.** Tamoxifen blocks the oestrogen receptor.
     E. **True.**
     F. **True.** After an initial release of LH.

33. A. **True.** 50% of patients receiving more than a total dose of
         400 mg/m².
     B. **False.** Azathioprine does not cause a peripheral neuropathy.
         The vinca alkaloids do.
     C. **True.**
     D. **True.**
     E. **False.** The nadir white count occurs 7–9 days after
         treatment.
     F. **True.** The risk is increased 40-fold after treatment for
         Hodgkin's disease.

34. A. **False.** The acid phosphatase is elevated in prostatic cancer.
     B. **True.**
     C. **True.**
     D. **True.** In 95% of cases.
     E. **False.** Although elevated in 65% of cases, CEA
         measurement is not sensitive or specific enough for use as a
         screening test.
     F. **True.**

35. Aetiological factors in cancer include:

A. β-Naphthylamine and bladder cancer.
B. Asbestos and mesothelioma.
C. Hepatitis A and hepatoma.
D. Herpes simplex 6 and cervical cancer.
E. Ultraviolet light and skin cancer.
F. *Aspergillus flavus* and hepatoma.

(Answers overleaf)

35. **A.** **True.**

B. **True.**

C. **False.** Hepatitis B infection is associated with development of hepatoma.

D. **False.** Herpes simplex 2 virus is associated with uterine cervix cancer.

E. **True.**

F. **True.**

9. Ageing and disease

36. The following physiological changes can be regarded as part of the normal ageing process:
A. Increased thirst in response to rises in plasma osmolality.
B. Reduced perception of cold conditions.
C. Reduced fasting plasma glucose level.
D. Cortical bone loss in postmenopausal women.
E. A slight increase in energy requirements.
F. Reduction in REM sleep.

37. In the elderly population of the UK:
A. The dramatic growth in the number of elderly people earlier this century was due mainly to improved health care of the elderly.
B. Life expectancy is greater for men than women.
C. The major cause of intellectual loss is arteriosclerotic dementia.
D. Most of the variation in mortality rates throughout the year is associated with changes in ambient temperature.
E. Parkinson's disease is the commonest cause of autonomic neuropathy.
F. Mortality is generally lowest when body weight is slightly below the ideal.

38. Causes of a dementia which might improve on treatment include the following:
A. Tertiary syphilis.
B. Iron deficiency anaemia.
C. Alzheimer's disease.
D. Depression.
E. Frontal meningioma.
F. Normal pressure (communicating) hydrocephalus.

(Answers overleaf)

36. A. False.   The elderly have a reduced sensation of thirst in response to rises in plasma osmolality.

    B. True.   They are less aware of discomfort in cold living conditions and this increases their vulnerability to hypothermia.

    C. False.   The mean fasting blood glucose level increases very slightly with advancing age.

    D. False.   There is loss of mainly trabecular bone, leading to vertebral and distal forearm fractures.

    E. False.   There is a marked decrease in energy requirements, mainly through physical illness and reduced physical activity, although healthy and active persons over 60 years of age have energy and nutrient requirements similar to those of a 30-year-old.

    F. False.   The pattern of REM sleep remains the same throughout adult life, although it may be reduced in the very old. Slow-wave sleep is reduced, and stage four sleep is almost completely absent.

37. A. False.   It was due largely to the reductions in infant mortality from infectious diseases, achieved around the turn of this century.

    B. False.   Life expectancy at birth is 72.8 years for males and 78.3 years for females.

    C. False.   It is senile dementia of the Alzheimer's type (Alzheimer's disease).

    D. True.   About 80% of the variation is due to a marked excess mortality during the cold winter months.

    E. False.   It is diabetes mellitus.

    F. False.   Mortality is generally lowest when body weight is slightly above the ideal.

38. A. True.

    B. False.   Vitamin B_{12} deficiency can cause a dementia which may respond to treatment.

    C. False.   There are claims to treatment that may slow down the rate of decline in intellectual function, but no treatment that can reverse the condition.

    D. True.

    E. True.

    F. True.

39. **In prescribing for the elderly:**
   A. Adverse drug reactions are more likely.
   B. The volume of distribution of lipid-soluble drugs is reduced.
   C. Temazepam is more suitable than lormetazepam as a hypnotic.
   D. Heminevrin is a suitable hypnotic.
   E. Cardiac sensitivity to propranolol increases with age.
   F. The dose of warfarin required to produce anticoagulation is reduced.

(Answers overleaf)

39. **A.** **True.** Two to three times more common, compared to people under the age of 60.

B. **False.** The increase in body fat in the elderly increases the volume of distribution.

C. **False.** The half-life of temazepam may be as long as 30 hours in the elderly, compared to 5–10 hours in young people; accumulation therefore occurs, which may result in daytime sedation and slowing of reaction times. The half-life of lormetazepam is prolonged up to 14 hours in the elderly, but accumulation does not occur with a nightly dose of 0.5 mg or 1.0 mg.

D. **True.** Its pharmacokinetics are virtually unaltered by age, and its short half-life of 3–4 hours means that accumulation does not occur.

E. **False.** It decreases.

F. **True.** The synthesis of vitamin K-dependent clotting factors is more sensitive to inhibition by warfarin in the elderly.

10. Psychological medicine

40. In psychotic depression:
A. Auditory hallucinations may be experienced.
B. Patients are often disorientated in time and place.
C. There is difficulty getting off to sleep.
D. Treatment with a tricyclic antidepressant is usually unhelpful.
E. There may be a family history of manic-depressive psychosis.
F. Diurnal rhythm of cortisol secretion may be abolished.

41. Anorexia nervosa:
A. Usually starts in the third decade.
B. Both sexes are affected equally.
C. Is fatal in up to 5% of cases.
D. May be associated with bulimia.
E. Is associated with hypogonadotrophic hypogonadism.
F. Causes loss of libido in males.

42. In patients with schizophrenia:
A. Auditory hallucinations in the first person are characteristic.
B. First-rank symptoms include thought insertion and broadcasting.
C. Deja vu phenomena are common.
D. An acute onset of the illness is associated with a more favourable prognosis.
E. A disturbance of mid-brain cholinergic pathways is postulated.
F. CT scanning of the brain is normal.

(Answers overleaf)

40. A. True. They are usually self-denigratory.
   B. False. Clear consciousness with full orientation is maintained, in contrast to organic psychosis.
   C. False. This is characteristic of neurotic depression; early morning wakening is characteristic of psychotic depression.
   D. False. Tricyclic antidepressants are the first line treatment in moderate *and* severe depression.
   E. True. There is a genetic predisposition, as shown by twin studies.
   F. True. Plasma cortisol may fail to suppress normally after administration of dexamethasone; this is sometimes useful diagnostically.

41. A. False. It usually starts in early or mid-adolescence.
   B. False. Some 90% of patients are female.
   C. True. About 5–10% die, poor prognosis being associated with later onset, 'atypical features', marked body image disturbance and self-induced vomiting.
   D. True. There is an overlap with bulimia nervosa, with binge–vomit cycles.
   E. True. Probably as a consequence of weight loss, rather than a primary endocrine disturbance.
   F. True. Male anorexics usually have severe disturbance of sexual identity.

42. A. False. The auditory hallucinations are characteristically in the third person, e.g. commentating on the patient's actions.
   B. True. These are known as 'passivity feelings'.
   C. False. They are not a feature, and are more suggestive of temporal lobe seizures.
   D. True. Other factors suggesting a better prognosis are: a clear precipitant, florid symptoms, marked mood change, previously good social adjustment and personality.
   E. False. The dopaminergic pathways are thought to be affected.
   F. False. In a subgroup of patients with no family history of schizophrenia, abnormalities may be seen on CT.

43. In suicide and parasuicide:

A. Suicide is commonest in young men.

B. Suicide is often an impulsive act.

C. The mode of death in suicide is usually violent.

D. Most people who commit suicide are suffering from psychiatric illness.

E. Personality disorder predisposes to repeated parasuicide.

F. Parasuicide is the commonest cause of an acute medical admission in women aged under 65.

44. In drug addiction and alcoholism:

A. It is a legal requirement to inform the Home Office of any patient suspected of being an opiate addict.

B. Any fully registered doctor in the United Kingdom can prescribe morphine for the maintenance of addiction.

C. Alcohol consumption per capita has decreased since 1950 in the United Kingdom.

D. The onset of confabulations in an alcoholic patient indicates irreversible brain damage.

E. Auditory hallucinations in the presence of clear consciousness can occur in alcoholics.

F. Amphetamine-induced psychosis persists for several months following withdrawal of the drug.

(Answers overleaf)

43. **A. True.** There has been a dramatic increase in suicide in young men between the ages of 18 and 35 over the past ten years.
    B. False. It is usually planned. Parasuicide is usually impulsive.
    C. True. Hanging, shooting and drowning are examples.
    D. True. About 90%, usually with depressive illness.
    E. True. As do alcohol and drug abuse.
    F. True. Parasuicide has reached epidemic proportions, with a four-fold incidence between 1963 and 1983. It is commonest in females aged 18–35.

44. **A. True.**
    B. False. A special licence is needed for maintenance, although any doctor can prescribe a morphine analogue such as methadone in a withdrawal crisis.
    C. False. There has been a 200% increase in consumption.
    D. False. This is Korsakoff syndrome and may fully reverse with vitamin treatment.
    E. True.
    F. False. Symptoms abate within two weeks of amphetamine withdrawal.

11. Infectious, tropical and parasitic diseases

45. Benzyl penicillin:
A. May be administered either parenterally or by mouth.
B. Has little activity against Gram-negative bacteria.
C. Acts by inhibition of bacterial protein synthesis.
D. Has a longer duration of action than procaine penicillin.
E. Is the drug of choice in meningococcal meningitis.
F. Is not active against *Listeria monocytogenes*.

46. The following are true of antifungal agents:
A. Amphotericin B is not absorbed from the intestine.
B. The dose of amphotericin B is limited by hepatic toxicity.
C. Flucytosine may be used alone in the treatment of systemic candidiasis.
D. Ketoconazole is effective treatment for oesophageal candidiasis.
E. Griseofulvin is deposited selectively in the dermis.
F. Fluconazole may be used to treat cryptococcal meningitis.

47. The following vaccines are of the live, attenuated type:
A. Diphtheria.
B. Measles, mumps, rubella (MMR).
C. Hepatitis B.
D. Oral polio.
E. Yellow fever.
F. Bacille Calmette–Guérin (BCG).

48. In Gram-negative septicaemia:
A. Endotoxin is a component of the bacterial cell wall.
B. Vascular permeability is increased.
C. Purpuric skin lesions are suggestive of *Haemophilus* infection.
D. Antibiotic therapy should be started once the causative organism has been isolated.
E. *Pseudomonas* infection usually responds to cefotaxime.
F. Corticosteroids should be prescribed if adult respiratory distress syndrome develops.

(Answers overleaf)

45. A. False. There is no oral preparation.
    B. True. However, it is active against *Neisseria*.
    C. False. It inhibits bacterial cell wall synthesis.
    D. False. Procaine penicillin is longer acting.
    E. True. However, resistant isolates have been reported in some parts of the world.
    F. False. There is good activity.

46. A. True. It has to be given intravenously or topically for oral candida.
    B. False. It is limited by renal and haemopoietic toxicity.
    C. False. Resistance develops rapidly if flucytosine is administered alone.
    D. True.
    E. False. It is deposited in keratin; this agent is used in severe dermatophyte infections.
    F. True. It is less toxic than amphotericin B but may not be as effective.

47. A. False. Toxoid.
    B. True. All three are live, attenuated.
    C. False. Purified or recombinant surface antigen.
    D. True.
    E. True. 17D strain virus.
    F. True.

48. A. True. It is the lipopolysaccharide component, especially lipid A.
    B. True.
    C. False. They are suggestive of meningococcaemia.
    D. False. Empiric therapy should be started immediately; it can be modified when the organism has been isolated.
    E. False. *Pseudomonas* is usually resistant to cefotaxime but sensitive to ceftazidime.
    F. False. They are of no proven benefit.

49. **The following diagnoses should be considered in a patient who presents with onset of fever 3 months after returning from the tropics:**
   A. Hepatitis A.
   B. Typhoid.
   C. Hepatitis B.
   D. *Plasmodium vivax* malaria.
   E. Dengue fever.
   F. Visceral leishmaniasis.

50. **The following organisms cause toxin-mediated diarrhoea and/or vomiting:**
   A. *Salmonella enteritidis.*
   B. *Vibrio cholerae.*
   C. *Staphylococcus.*
   D. *Bacillus cereus.*
   E. Enteropathogenic *Escherichia coli.*
   F. *Cryptosporidium.*

51. **In varicella zoster virus infection:**
   A. The incubation period of chickenpox is 1–2 weeks.
   B. The rash of chickenpox usually starts on the face.
   C. The severity of chickenpox is increased after puberty.
   D. Shingles results from reactivation of the virus in anterior horn cells of the spinal cord.
   E. Fetal damage can occur during the third trimester of pregnancy as a result of placental passage of the virus.
   F. Chickenpox may be complicated by bleeding due to thrombocytopenia.

52. **The following are true of cytomegalovirus (CMV):**
   A. The majority of infections are asymptomatic.
   B. It is a single-stranded RNA virus.
   C. Primary infection may cause generalised lymphadenopathy with a positive Monospot test.
   D. Retinitis is the most frequent manifestation in AIDS patients.
   E. The virus may be cultured from the urine in active infection.
   F. Pneumonitis is best treated with acyclovir.

(Answers overleaf)

49. A. False. The incubation period is 2–6 weeks.
   B. False. The incubation period is 1–3 weeks.
   C. True. The incubation period is up to 6 months.
   D. True. The latent liver hypnozoites can cause relapse months or years after infection.
   E. False. The incubation period is about one week.
   F. True. The incubation period is from 2 weeks to 2 years.

50. A. False. It invades the gut mucosa.
   B. True. Exotoxin binds to jejunal enterocytes and activates cAMP.
   C. True. Preformed enterotoxins cause rapid-onset diarrhoea and vomiting.
   D. True. Heat-stable toxin is either ingested with food or released in the intestine by ingested organisms.
   E. False. The mechanism is uncertain.
   F. False. It invades the enterocytes.

51. A. False. It is 15–18 days.
   B. False. It starts on the trunk then spreads to face and limbs.
   C. True. It is usually a mild illness in children.
   D. False. The virus is reactivated in the dorsal root ganglia.
   E. False. The virus can cross the placenta during the first 20 weeks of pregnancy.
   F. True. Consumptive coagulopathy may also occur.

52. A. True. However, this is not the case in immunocompromised subjects.
   B. False. It is a double-stranded DNA virus (herpes virus).
   C. False. The Monospot is negative.
   D. True. Oral and oesophageal ulceration, colitis and, rarely, pneumonitis may also occur.
   E. True.
   F. False. Ganciclovir and foscarnet are more active against CMV.

53. In a child presenting with fever and rash, the following favour the diagnosis of measles:

A. Lymphadenopathy confined to the occipital and posterior cervical regions.

B. Lack of constitutional symptoms.

C. Spots appearing first behind the ears.

D. Discrete, pale macules which do not coalesce.

E. Widespread crackles on chest auscultation.

F. Palatal petechiae.

54. In rubella infection:

A. The incubation period is about 2 weeks.

B. The rash persists for at least a week in most cases.

C. Arthritis is most common in young men.

D. Specific antibody is detectable by the haemagglutination inhibition test within a week of exposure.

E. In pregnancy the risk to the fetus is greatest in the first month.

F. Atrial septal defect is the most common cardiac lesion in the congenital form.

55. The following are true of Chlamydia:

A. They are bacteria which contain both DNA and RNA.

B. They are obligate intracellular pathogens.

C. *Chl. psittaci* infection is best treated with ampicillin.

D. *Chl. trachomatis* causes granuloma inguinale.

E. They may be seen on Gram stain of urethral smears in non-specific genital infection.

F. Chronic trachoma infection leads to entropion.

56. In typhoid (enteric fever):

A. The incubation period is usually less than one week.

B. Dry cough is a common early feature.

C. Diarrhoea is usual in the first week.

D. The diagnosis is best made using the Widal test.

E. Relapse occurs in 15% cases, despite appropriate antibiotic treatment.

F. A one week course of ciprofloxacin is effective treatment.

(Answers overleaf)

53. **A.** **False.** Generalised lymphadenopathy in measles, occipital and posterior cervical in rubella.
   B. **False.** Marked constitutional upset is ususal.
   C. **True.** They occur also on the forehead, spreading to the face and then to the trunk and limbs.
   D. **False.** Red macules which enlarge and coalesce to form blotches.
   E. **True.** Respiratory symptoms and signs are common.
   F. **False.** Diffuse erythema of the buccal mucosa and Koplik's spots are characteristic; palatal petechiae are common in rubella.

54. **A.** **True.** It is 14–16 days.
   B. **False.** It persists for up to 4 days.
   C. **False.** It is most common in young women.
   D. **False.** It is detectable 14–16 days after infection, at the time of the onset of clinical illness.
   E. **True.** Over 50% fetuses are affected at this stage.
   F. **False.** Patent ductus arteriosus, with or without pulmonary stenosis, is the most common cardiac lesion in congenital rubella.

55. **A.** **True.** Unlike viruses, which contain either DNA or RNA.
   B. **True.** They are unable to replicate extracellularly.
   C. **False.** Tetracyclines are the treatment of choice.
   D. **False.** It causes lymphogranuloma venereum, non-specific genital infection and trachoma.
   E. **False.** Gram stain shows excess polymorphs but no organisms.
   F. **True.** This is due to inflammation leading to fibrosis.

56. **A.** **False.** It is 1–3 weeks.
   B. **True.**
   C. **False.** Constipation is followed by diarrhoea in the third week.
   D. **False.** Culture organisms from blood, urine or stool; the Widal test for agglutinating antibody is not useful.
   E. **True.**
   F. **False.** Ciprofloxacin is effective, but treatment should continue for at least 2 weeks in total, or one week after defervescence.

57. Whooping cough:
A. Is transmitted from person to person by droplet.
B. Is most common in children over the age of 5 years.
C. Usually causes a neutrophilia in the peripheral blood.
D. Responds well to treatment with erythromycin.
E. Vaccination is only 80% effective in preventing the disease.
F. May be complicated by convulsions.

58. In leprosy:
A. The causative organism may be cultured *in vitro* from skin.
B. Most infections are asymptomatic.
C. The lepromin test is positive in the tuberculoid form.
D. The lepromatous form is characterised by anaesthetic skin lesions.
E. The treatment of choice is a combination of dapsone and isoniazid.
F. The incidence is reduced by BCG vaccination.

59. The following diseases are caused by spirochaetes:
A. Yaws.
B. Louse-borne relapsing fever.
C. Q fever.
D. Lyme disease.
E. Pinta.
F. Sporotrichosis.

60. Giardiasis:
A. Is characterised by bloody diarrhoea.
B. May be transmitted from person to person.
C. Is a frequent cause of diarrhoea in patients with AIDS.
D. May present as failure to thrive in childhood.
E. May be treated by a single dose of tinidazole.
F. May be diagnosed by finding cysts in jejunal juice.

(Answers overleaf)

57. **A. True.**
    B. False. It is most common under the age of 5, but it may occur at any age.
    C. False. It usually causes lymphocytosis.
    D. False. The organism is sensitive, but treatment has little effect on the course of the illness.
    E. True. However, it may reduce the severity if it does not prevent the disease completely.
    F. True. Coughing spasms can cause cerebral hypoxia.

58. **A. False.** *Mycobacterium leprae* may be seen on Ziehl–Neelsen staining but cannot be cultured *in vitro*.
    B. True. The outcome of infection depends on the host's immune response.
    C. True. It indicates delayed type hypersensitivity to the organism.
    D. False. The tuberculoid form is characterised by such lesions.
    E. False. Dapsone and rifampicin, with or without clofazimine, is the treatment of choice.
    F. True.

59. **A. True.** The causal agent is *Treponema pertenue*.
    B. True. The causal agent is *Borrelia recurrentis*.
    C. False. This disease is caused by *Coxiella burnetii* (rickettsial infection).
    D. True. The causal agent is *Borrelia burgdorferi*.
    E. True. The causal agent is *Treponema carateum*.
    F. False. This disease is caused by *Sporothrix schenckii* (fungal infection).

60. **A. False.** The stools are yellow and offensive, without blood.
    B. True. This is especially the case in children and male homosexuals.
    C. False. It is not a major cause.
    D. True. Chronic *Giardia* infection leads to malabsorption.
    E. True. This is an alternative to metronidazole, which requires at least 3 doses.
    F. False. Diagnosis requires the finding of trophozoites.

61. Infection with *Entamoeba histolytica*:

A. Is almost always symptomatic.

B. Is more common in adults than children.

C. Is spread by ingestion of the trophozoites by the faecal–oral route.

D. May present as an abdominal mass.

E. Should be treated with metronidazole to eradicate luminal cysts.

F. Is associated with positive serological tests in 95% of cases of dysentery.

62. The following are true of trypanosomiasis:

A. *T. gambiense* infection causes sleeping sickness.

B. Man is the reservoir for *T. rhodesiense*.

C. The tsetse fly is the insect vector for *T. cruzi*.

D. The diagnosis of *T. cruzi* infection can be made only by serology.

E. Suramin is ineffective for the treatment of CNS involvement in *T. rhodesiense* infection.

F. Hepatosplenomegaly is a feature of acute Chagas' disease.

63. In toxoplasmosis:

A. The dog is the definitive host for the parasite.

B. Transmission to man may occur by eating undercooked meat.

C. Asymptomatic infection is rare.

D. The diagnosis is made by isolation of the parasite in stool.

E. Congenital infection may result from maternal infection during the third trimester of pregnancy.

F. Reactivation of latent infection in immunosuppressed patients is most commonly within the brain.

64. The following are true of malaria:

A. Sporozoites are transmitted to man by the bite of the *Anopheles* mosquito.

B. *Pl. vivax* has no hypnozoite form.

C. *Pl. falciparum* infection may lead to renal failure.

D. *Pl. ovale* infection is always chloroquine sensitive.

E. Focal neurological deficit is rare in cerebral malaria.

F. Prophylaxis with pyrimethamine is recommended for travel to areas with a low risk of chloroquine resistance.

(Answers overleaf)

61. A. False. It is commonly an asymptomatic, non-invasive infection.
   B. True.
   C. False. It is spread by the ingestion of cysts.
   D. True. It may present as an 'amoeboma'—a mass of granulation tissue containing few amoebae.
   E. False. Metronidazole kills invasive trophozoites, but diloxanide furoate is required to eradicate luminal cysts.
   F. False. Serology is positive in only about 60% of cases of dysentery.

62. A. True. *T. rhodesiense* also causes the disease.
   B. False. Various wild mammals form the reservoir; man is an incidental host (unlike *T. gambiense*).
   C. False. Reduviid bugs are the vectors; tsetse flies transmit African trypanosomiasis.
   D. False. Parasites may be seen in peripheral blood and CSF in acute infection.
   E. True. Melarsoprol is used if there is CNS involvement; suramin does not cross the blood–brain barrier.
   F. True. Fever, lymphadenopathy and cardiac involvement are also features.

63. A. False. The cat is the definitive host.
   B. True. Pigs or sheep may act as intermediate hosts.
   C. False. Asymptomatic infection is common, especially in immunocompetent adults.
   D. False. It is made by serology.
   E. True.
   F. True. It often presents as mass lesions.

64. A. True.
   B. False. *Plasmodium falciparum* has no hypnozoite form.
   C. True. Renal failure is usually due to acute tubular necrosis, with or without severe haemolysis.
   D. True.
   E. True. Altered consciousness and convulsions are typical manifestations.
   F. False. Chloroquine or proguanil is recommended.

65. Causes of a peripheral blood eosinophilia include:

A. Visceral larva migrans (toxocariasis).
B. Giardiasis.
C. Malaria.
D. *Loa loa*.
E. Hydatid disease.
F. *Enterobius vermicularis* (threadworm).

66. In filarial infection:

A. Transmission from person to person is by insect bite.
B. *Onchocerca volvulus* infection may cause corneal scarring.
C. Diethylcarbamazine is the drug of choice in *W. bancrofti* infection.
D. Calabar swellings are a feature of lymphatic filariasis.
E. Adult worms develop from infective larvae in about 2 weeks.
F. *Loa loa* occurs predominantly in South America.

67. Schistosoma:

A. Are intestinal nematodes.
B. Eggs are passed in urine or stool.
C. *S. mansoni* infection occurs predominantly in the Far East.
D. *S. mansoni* infection may lead to portal hypertension.
E. *S. haematobium* infection rarely presents with haematuria.
F. Infection should be treated with mebendazole.

(Answers overleaf)

65. A. **True.** Disseminated *Toxocara* larvae.
    B. **False.**
    C. **False.**
    D. **True.** Filarial infection.
    E. **True.** *Echinococcus granulosus* (dog tapeworm).
    F. **False.**

66. A. **True.** Microfilariae migrate out of the insect's mouth and enter the skin.
    B. **True.** It may lead to blindness.
    C. **True.** It is more effective against microfilariae than adult worms.
    D. **False.** These are transient soft tissue swellings seen in *Loa loa*.
    E. **False.** They develop in about 6 months.
    F. **False.** The disease occurs predominantly in West and Central Africa.

67. A. **False.** They are trematodes.
    B. **True.**
    C. **False.** *S. mansoni* occurs in South America and Africa; *S. japonicum* is found in the Far East.
    D. **True.** Liver granulomas obstruct portal blood flow and lead to periportal fibrosis.
    E. **False.** Haematuria (especially terminal) is common.
    F. **False.** Praziquantel, oxamniquine or metrifonate should be used for treatment.

12. Skin disease

68. Psoriasis:
A. Demonstrates the Koebner phenomenon in response to trauma.
B. Epidermal turnover is reduced.
C. May be precipitated by streptococcal pharyngitis.
D. Is not itchy.
E. May be precipitated by exposure to UV radiation.
F. Is associated with HLA-CW6.

69. In the treatment of psoriasis:
A. Oral therapy with antimitotics is usually required.
B. Discoid lesions respond poorly to topical tar and dithranol.
C. Nail dystrophy responds well to topical therapy with tar.
D. Methotrexate therapy may be complicated by hepatic fibrosis.
E. Photochemotherapy (PUVA) is associated with an increased risk of non-melanoma skin cancer.
F. Calcipotriol is a vitamin A analogue useful in topical treatment.

70. The following are true about eczema:
A. The rash is typically itchy and red.
B. Patch testing is useful in detecting the cause of exogenous eczema.
C. The onset of exogenous eczema is within the first 3 months of life.
D. Atopic eczema is associated with asthma.
E. May start with a herald patch.
F. Nickel jewellery is a common sensitiser.

(Answers overleaf)

68. A. **True.**
    B. **False.** Epidermal turnover is increased to 5–7 days compared to 30–45 days.
    C. **True.** Typically guttate psoriasis.
    D. **False.** It is often itchy.
    E. **True.**
    F. **True.** The risk is increased 5–10-fold.

69. A. **False.** Most patients can be treated successfully with topical agents.
    B. **False.** They respond well.
    C. **False.** There is a poor response.
    D. **True.** May be diagnosed on liver biopsy.
    E. **True.**
    F. **False.** Calcipotriol is a topical vitamin D analogue.

70. A. **True.**
    B. **True.**
    C. **False.** The onset of endogenous eczema is often within the first 3 months of life.
    D. **True.**
    E. **False.** A feature of pityriasis rosea.
    F. **True.**

71. The following are true about urticaria:

A. The rash is characteristically a raised weal which does not itch.
B. Lasts more than 24 hours.
C. When chronic may be due to IgG autoantibodies against IgE.
D. Occurs as a result of mast cell degranulation and release of histamine.
E. Hereditary angio-oedema is due to a deficiency of C1 esterase.
F. Angio-oedema occurs in the subcutaneous tissue.

72. Causes of erythema nodosum include:

A. Sarcoidosis.
B. Reiter's syndrome.
C. Sulphonamides.
D. Oral contraceptive pill.
E. Wegener's granulomatosis.
F. Leprosy.

73. Scabies:

A. Is caused by *Sarcoptes scabiei*.
B. The female mite is visible to the naked eye.
C. Burrows are typically seen on the wrists.
D. Itching occurs at the same time as the initial attack.
E. Can be treated with malathion.
F. Excoriation can occur.

74. Features of Henoch–Schönlein purpura include:

A. Arthralgia.
B. Abdominal pain.
C. Palpable purpura chiefly on the buttocks and extensor surfaces of the limbs.
D. Haematuria.
E. Occurs predominantly in adults.
F. Leucocytoclastic vasculitis with IgA deposition.

(Answers overleaf)

71. A. **False.** Itching is often severe.
    B. **False.** Rarely last more than 24 hours.
    C. **True.**
    D. **True.**
    E. **False.** It is due to a deficiency of C1 esterase inhibitor.
    F. **True.**

72. A. **True.**
    B. **False.**
    C. **True.**
    D. **True.**
    E. **False.**
    F. **False.** Clinically and histologically different from erythema nodosum.

73. A. **True.**
    B. **True.**
    C. **True.**
    D. **False.** Two months later.
    E. **True.**
    F. **True.**

74. A. **True.**
    B. **True.**
    C. **True.** Typical distribution.
    D. **True.**
    E. **False.** It is rare in adults.
    F. **True.** The characteristic histological appearance.

75. **Typical features of pemphigus vulgaris include:**
    A. Subepidermal blisters.
    B. Nikolsky's sign.
    C. Acantholysis.
    D. Mucous membrane involvement.
    E. Presence of antibodies against desmoglein.
    F. Blisters which remain intact for several days.

76. **Recognised features of dermatitis herpetiformis include:**
    A. Association with HLA-B8.
    B. IgG deposition in unaffected skin.
    C. Subtotal villous atrophy on jejunal biopsy.
    D. Itchiness.
    E. Intra-epidermal blisters.
    F. Response to dapsone.

77. **Typical features of malignant melanoma:**
    A. Association with chronic sun damage.
    B. Rising incidence.
    C. Should be suspected in an enlarging itchy pigmented lesion.
    D. Prognosis is poor.
    E. May arise from previously normal-looking skin.
    F. May develop from a rodent ulcer.

78. **The following are true about sunlight:**
    A. Ultraviolet B (UVB) has a shorter wavelength than ultraviolet A (UVA).
    B. UVB is responsible for acute sunburn.
    C. UVA is filtered out by ordinary glass windows.
    D. UV light converts 7-dihydrocholesterol to pre-vitamin D_3.
    E. Photosensitivity occurs in acute intermittent porphyria.
    F. Polymorphic light eruption is itchy.

79. **Typical features of vitiligo include:**
    A. Loss of melanocytes from the basal layer of the epidermis.
    B. Scaling.
    C. Anaesthesia.
    D. Clear demarcation of patches.
    E. Increased frequency of non-organic-specific autoimmune disease.
    F. Yellow fluorescence under Wood's light.

(Answers overleaf)

75. **A. False.** A feature of bullous pemphigoid, the blisters of pemphigus are intra-epidermal.
    B. True. Sideways pressure on the skin produces new blisters.
    C. True.
    D. True.
    E. True.
    F. False. They are very fragile. The blisters of pemphigoid last for several days.

76. **A. True.**
    B. False. IgA is deposited.
    C. True. The histological features of coeliac disease.
    D. True.
    E. False. The blisters are subepidermal blisters.
    F. True. The response may be dramatic.

77. **A. False.** Associated with short bursts of sun exposure.
    B. True.
    C. True.
    D. False. Prognosis depends on depth of invasion. Superficial lesions can be completely excised.
    E. True.
    F. False. Rodent ulcers are basal cell carcinomas.

78. **A. True.** UVA 320–400 nm, UVB 290–320 nm, UVC 200–290 nm.
    B. True.
    C. False. UVB is filtered by ordinary glass.
    D. True.
    E. False. This is the only type of porphyria in which photosensitivity is not a feature.
    F. True.

79. **A. True.**
    B. False. Scaling is not a feature.
    C. False. A feature of leprosy.
    D. True.
    E. False. It is more frequently associated with the organ-specific autoimmune diseases.
    F. False. Pityriasis versicolor fluoresces yellow, vitiligo appears white.

13. AIDS and genitourinary medicine

80. Human immunodeficiency virus (HIV):
- **A.** Is a double-stranded, non-enveloped RNA virus.
- **B.** Is not known to be transmitted by saliva.
- **C.** Leads to progressive depletion of CD8 cytotoxic lymphocytes.
- **D.** Infection is commonly asymptomatic in the first 5 years.
- **E.** Infection leads to raised immunoglobulin levels.
- **F.** May be transmitted by breast-feeding.

81. In HIV infection:
- **A.** *Toxoplasma* is the most frequent cause of meningitis.
- **B.** Kaposi's sarcoma is more common amongst homosexuals than other groups.
- **C.** Cytomegalovirus is a common cause of pneumonia.
- **D.** *Cryptococcus* is the commonest cause of diarrhoea.
- **E.** Pharyngitis is a feature of the acute seroconversion illness.
- **F.** Zidovudine inhibits the viral protease enzyme.

82. *Pneumocystis carinii* pneumonia:
- **A.** Occurs only in patients with AIDS.
- **B.** Is characterised by a cough productive of purulent sputum.
- **C.** Is associated with bilateral fine infiltrates on chest X-ray.
- **D.** Often causes profound hypercapnia.
- **E.** Is diagnosed by sputum culture.
- **F.** Is exacerbated by administration of corticosteroids.

80. A. False. It is a single-stranded RNA, enveloped retrovirus.
   B. True. However, the virus can be cultured from saliva (and tears).
   C. False. It depletes CD4 helper lymphocytes.
   D. True. The mean time to develop AIDS is 8–10 years.
   E. True. Polyclonal B cell activation, but poor specific antibody responses.
   F. True.

81. A. False. *Cryptococcus neoformans* is the most frequent cause; *Toxoplasma* causes encephalitis with mass lesions within the brain.
   B. True. It is believed to be caused by a newly identified herpes virus (KSHV).
   C. False. Cytomegalovirus is commonly seen in broncho-alveolar lavage fluid but it rarely causes pneumonia.
   D. False. *Cryptosporidium* is the commonest pathogen isolated.
   E. True. Fever, rash, lymphadenopathy and arthralgia also occur.
   F. False. It inhibits viral reverse transcriptase.

82. A. False. It also occurs in other immunocompromised patients and in premature infants.
   B. False. There is usually a dry cough and dyspnoea.
   C. True. However, it may be normal in the early stages.
   D. False. Hypoxaemia is common.
   E. False. The organism may be identified by silver stain or immunofluorescence in induced sputum or broncho-alveolar lavage fluid.
   F. False. The addition of steroids to antibiotics is beneficial in severe infection.

83. *Neisseria gonorrhoeae* (gonococcus):
    A. Is a Gram-negative bacillus.
    B. Infection is usually asymptomatic in females.
    C. Infection is best diagnosed by dark-ground microscopy of smears.
    D. Infection may be treated with high-dose cotrimoxazole.
    E. Disseminated infection is more common in women than in men.
    F. Infection has an incubation period of around 6–8 weeks.

84. **The following are true of syphilis:**
    A. The primary chancre is usually painless.
    B. Systemic upset is rare in the secondary stage.
    C. The VDRL test is usually negative in the secondary stage.
    D. Sexual transmission is rare during the latent phase.
    E. A vesicular rash is a feature of early congenital infection.
    F. The Jarisch–Herxheimer reaction is seen most commonly during treatment in the primary stage.

(Answers overleaf)

83. A. **False.** It is a Gram-negative coccus.
    B. **True.** However, it may cause vaginal discharge, dysuria and abdominal pain.
    C. **False.** It is best diagnosed by Gram stain of smears and culture (dark-ground microscopy is used to look for spirochaetes).
    D. **True.** Cotrimoxazole may be used in penicillin-allergic subjects.
    E. **True.**
    F. **False.** The incubation period is 2–7 days.

84. A. **True.**
    B. **False.** Systemic upset with fever is common.
    C. **False.** It is almost always positive at high titre.
    D. **True.** However, feto-maternal transmission may occur.
    E. **True.** It is not seen in adults.
    F. **False.** It is most common in the secondary stage.

14. Cardiovascular disease

85. In the normal heart:
A. Lactate is metabolised to pyruvate.
B. The upstroke of the cardiac action potential corresponds to an influx of sodium ions.
C. The venous return to the heart falls during inspiration.
D. Preload is the force against which the myocardium contracts.
E. Isovolumic ventricular contraction terminates when the mitral valve opens.
F. Myocardial wall tension in diastole is inversely proportional to ventricular diameter.

86. The following statements are correct:
A. Pericardial pain may be relieved by leaning forwards.
B. The pain from a dissecting aortic aneurysm often radiates through to the back.
C. Pulmonary venous hypertension can cause a dry cough.
D. Oesophageal spasm may be relieved by GTN spray.
E. Syncope during exertion usually has a non-cardiac cause.
F. Significant myocardial ischaemia is invariably accompanied by chest discomfort.

87. Classical abnormalities of the jugular venous pressure (JVP) waveform include:
A. Absent 'a' waves in atrial fibrillation.
B. Cannon 'a' waves in complete heart block.
C. Large 'v' waves in pulmonary hypertension.
D. Giant 'a' waves in tricuspid regurgitation.
E. A slow 'y' descent in tricuspid stenosis.
F. A rapid 'x' descent in pericardial tamponade.

(Answers overleaf)

85. **A.** **True.**
    B. **True.**
    C. **False.** The fall in intrathoracic preesure during inspiration augments venous return.
    D. **False.** This definition refers to the afterload. Preload is the myocardial fibre length at which contraction begins.
    E. **False.** Aortic valve opening terminates isovolumic contraction.
    F. **False.** The Law of Laplace states that:

$$\text{tension} = \text{distending pressure} \times \frac{\text{vessel radius}}{2 \times \text{wall thickness}}.$$

86. **A.** **True.**
    B. **True.**
    C. **True.** It can also cause wheezing ('cardiac asthma').
    D. **True.** The pain often follows the path of the dissection.
    E. **True.**
    F. **False.** Continuous ambulatory cardiac monitoring has shown that some episodes of myocardial ischaemia are 'silent'.

87. **A.** **True.** The 'a' wave is produced by atrial systole.
    B. **True.** These occur when the atrium contacts against a closed tricuspid valve.
    C. **False.** The 'v' wave is produced by ventricular systole. Large 'v' waves are seen in tricuspid regurgitation.
    D. **False.** Giant 'a' waves are seen in pulmonary hypertension.
    E. **True.**
    F. **True.**

88. In the auscultation of the heart:
A. The first heart sound immediately follows the carotid pulse upstroke.
B. The aortic component of the second sound occurs before the pulmonary.
C. Expiration increases the split of the second sound.
D. A loud opening snap occurs in diastole in mitral stenosis.
E. A fourth heart sound coincides with atrial systole.
F. A mid-diastolic click occurs in mitral valve prolapse.

89. Regarding the electrocardiogram:
A. The standard paper speed is 25 mm/min.
B. Standard lead III is at 90° to lead I.
C. The PR interval is measured from the end of the P wave to the peak of the R wave.
D. A QRS duration of > 0.12 seconds indicates bundle branch block.
E. A right bundle branch block may be a normal finding.
F. A mean frontal axis of +170°, indicates right axis deviation.

90. In cardiac failure:
A. The 5-year mortality is 50%.
B. Paraquat poisoning may precipitate acute pulmonary oedema.
C. Diamorphine is contraindicated in the treatment of acute pulmonary oedema.
D. Renin levels may be high.
E. Patients are usually hypoxic.
F. Treatment with ACE inhibitors prolongs survival.

(Answers overleaf)

88. **A.** **False.** The first heart sound precedes the carotid pulse upstroke and signals the beginning of systole.
    B. **True.** Prolongation of left ventricular ejection (e.g. severe aortic stenosis) can reverse this.
    C. **False.** Inspiration increases the split by increasing right-sided filling and therefore right-sided ejection time.
    D. **True.** Produced by the sudden, forceful opening of the tethered valve cusps.
    E. **True.** This occurs with increasing ventricular filling pressures.
    F. **False.** The click is mid-systolic and may be followed by a murmur of mitral regurgitation.

89. **A.** **False.** Standard paper speed is 25 mm/s.
    B. **False.** It is at 120° to lead I.
    C. **False.** The interval is measured from the start of the P wave.
    D. **True.**
    E. **True.**
    F. **True.** An axis greater than +120°, indicates right axis deviation.

90. **A.** **True.**
    B. **True.** As can overtransfusion, shock lung in septicaemia, aspiration of gastric contents and inhalation of certain toxic fumes.
    C. **False.**
    D. **True.** As a result of reduced afferent renal perfusion pressure.
    E. **True.** Hypoxia is common due to (1) a reduction in gas exchange, due to congested lungs, and (2) a fall in cardiac output which reduces mixed venous oxygen tension.
    F. **True.** But only by an average of 6 months.

91. **In heart block:**
    A. A PR interval of 0.18 seconds indicates first degree block.
    B. Cannon waves are seen in first degree block.
    C. Intermittent, unheralded failure of P wave conduction occurs in Mobitz type II block.
    D. In third degree block the QRS complexes are always abnormally widened.
    E. Mobitz type I block occurring during myocardial infarction requires a prophylactic pacing wire.
    F. In patients with complete heart block following anterior myocardial infarction the prognosis is good.

92. **In a patient with a broad complex tachycardia the following features favour an aberrant supraventricular rhythm from ventricular rhythm:**
    A. Duration of the QRS complex >160 milliseconds.
    B. Similar QRS morphology, not resembling bundle branch block, in the anterior chest leads.
    C. Independent P wave activity.
    D. The presence of fusion beats.
    E. The maintenance of a normal blood pressure.
    F. The presence of an underlying cardiomyopathy.

93. **In the treatment of tachyarrhythmias:**
    A. The immediate treatment of ventricular fibrillation is DC cardioversion.
    B. DC cardioversion is often effective in the treatment of atrial flutter.
    C. A combination of intravenous verapamil and a beta-blocker is effective in paroxysmal atrial tachycardia.
    D. Current digoxin treatment is an absolute contraindication to DC cardioversion.
    E. Flecainide is effective in the treatment of the Wolff–Parkinson–White syndrome.
    F. Digoxin can be used to treat atrial fibrillation in the Wolff–Parkinson–White syndrome.

(Answers overleaf)

91. A. False. Greater than 0.20 seconds.
 B. False. Seen in complete heart block where the atrium contracts against a closed tricuspid valve.
 C. True. A progressive increase is seen in Mobitz type I block.
 D. False. The block may be within the AV node, producing a narrow complex escape rhythm originating in the lower node or His bundle.
 E. False. This is generally a benign arrhythmia.
 F. False. Complete heart block in anterior myocardial infarction indicates very extensive cardiac damage.

92. A. False. Very broad complexes almost always indicate ventricular tachycardia (VT).
 B. False. Bizarre, concordant complexes favour VT.
 C. False. Diagnostic of VT.
 D. False. The fusion of a normal sinus beat with the abnormal ventricular complex is diagnostic of VT.
 E. False. VT can be surprisingly well tolerated.
 F. False. Any history of myocardial disease favours VT.

93. A. True. Cardiac output is invariably lost.
 B. True. Usually only a 25–50 J shock is needed.
 C. False. Combined intravenous therapy should be avoided. DC conversion is safer if single agents fail to restore sinus rhythm.
 D. False. Cardioversion is hazardous only in digoxin toxicity.
 E. True. Flecainide may increase mortality in post-infarct patients with ventricular arrhythmias.
 F. False. It may induce a very rapid ventricular rate by enhancing conduction through the aberrant pathway.

94. In cardiopulmonary resuscitation (CPR):

A. External cardiac massage should be performed at a rate of 30 compressions/minute.

B. A single-handed resuscitator should provide 15 chest compressions for every two mouth-to-mouth breaths.

C. Adrenaline may be given via an endotracheal tube.

D. Sodium bicarbonate should be given routinely given after 5 minutes of CPR.

E. Atropine is not used routinely in the treatment of asystole.

F. Lignocaine may cause CNS toxicity.

95. In mitral stenosis:

A. The stenosis is usually congenital.

B. There is a male preponderance.

C. Secondary tricuspid incompetence may develop.

D. The opening snap occurs close to the aortic second heart sound in severe stenosis.

E. The presystolic murmur is absent in patients in atrial fibrillation.

F. Balloon mitral valvotomy should not be performed if the valve is heavily calcified.

96. Mitral regurgitation has a recognised association with:

A. Acute myocardial infarction.

B. Ostium primum atrial septal defect.

C. Systemic lupus erythematosus.

D. Syphilis.

E. Marfan's syndrome.

F. Blunt chest trauma.

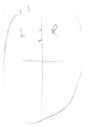

(Answers overleaf)

94. **A.** **False.** The UK Resuscitation Council recommends 60–80 compressions/minute.
    B. **True.** The ratio should be 5:1 if two people are available.
    C. **True.** Adrenaline can be given intravenously (1mg) or via an endotracheal tube (2mg).
    D. **False.** Only used in established acidosis, otherwise bicarbonate administration may worsen intracellular acidosis.
    E. **False.** A single bolus of 3mg i.v. should be given.
    F. **True.**

95. **A.** **False.** Mitral stenosis is almost always due to rheumatic heart disease; congenital stenosis is rare.
    B. **False.** It is commoner in women.
    C. **True.** Due to pulmonary hypertension.
    D. **True.**
    E. **True.** The presystolic murmur is due to turbulent flow through the stenosed valve during atrial contraction.
    F. **True.**

96. **A.** **True.** Acute inferior MI is associated with papillary muscle dysfunction and with papillary muscle rupture.
    B. **False.** Typically associated with ostium primum defects.
    C. **True.** As part of Libman-Sacks endocarditis.
    D. **True.** Associated with the ascending aortic aneurysm of quaternary syphilis.
    E. **True.** And with other collagen disorders.
    F. **True.** e.g. steering wheel injury during a road traffic accident.

97. The following statements are correct:

A. Few patients with bicuspid aortic valves ever develop significant aortic valve disease.

B. The murmur of aortic regurgitation is accentuated by expiration.

C. Aortic regurgitation is associated with ankylosing spondylitis.

D. A normal ECG virtually excludes significant aortic stenosis.

E. In aortic stenosis, the loudness of the murmur is proportional to the severity of the stenosis.

F. In aortic valve disease, angina can occur in the absence of any significant coronary artery disease.

98. Regarding congenital heart disease:

A. Ventricular septal defect is the most common lesion in livebirths.

B. Persistent ductus arteriosus (PDA) can occur as a result of maternal influenza virus infection in pregnancy.

C. Turner's syndrome is associated with coarctation of the aorta.

D. Atrial septal defect (ASD) is one of the principal features of Fallot's tetralogy.

E. The ostium primum defect is the most common form of ASD.

F. Patients with Epstein's anomaly of the tricuspid valve are seldom cyanosed.

99. The following are true of atrial septal defects (ASDs):

A. There is a well-recognised association with Down's syndrome.

B. Wide fixed splitting of the first heart sound is typical.

C. Classically, there is a loud systolic murmur with a thrill at the lower left sternal edge.

D. The Eisenmenger syndrome is associated with cyanosis.

E. A sinus venosus defect is frequently associated with anomalous pulmonary venous drainage.

F. The ECG in an ostium secundum defect usually shows left axis deviation.

(Answers overleaf)

97. A. False. Two thirds develop some form of aortic valve disease.
   B. True. Since LV output is increased.
   C. True. AR is also associated with other seronegative arthritides.
   D. True.
   E. False. Loudness of the murmur is a poor index of severity: the murmur may be absent in heart failure.
   F. True. Angina can be a feature of both AS and AR in the presence of normal coronary arteries, although coronary artery disease frequently co-exists in older patients.

98. A. False. ASD is the most common congenital heart defect in livebirths, representing 30% of all cases; VSD represents 9%.
   B. False. Congenital rubella infection is associated with PDA, ASD and pulmonary stenosis.
   C. True. And is also associated with pulmonary stenosis and bicuspid aortic valve.
   D. False. Fallot's consist of a VSD, pulmonary stenosis, an overriding aorta and right ventricular hypertrophy.
   E. False. The secundum defect is most common.
   F. False. Ebstein's anomaly is typically cyanotic.

99. A. True.
   B. False. Wide fixed splitting of the *second* heart sound is typical.
   C. False. This would suggest a VSD.
   D. True. Due to right-to-left shunting.
   E. True.
   F. True. The ECG in an ostium secundum defect typically shows right bundle branch block. Conversely, the ECG in a primum defect typically shows left bundle branch block.

100. Coarctation of the aorta:

  A. Is more common in men.
  B. Is associated with aortic dissection.
  C. Usually occurs proximal to the left subclavian artery.
  D. Surgical correction should be avoided in childhood.
  E. May produce a weak left radial pulse.
  F. Is associated with bicuspid aortic valves.

101. In the coronary circulation:

  A. Coronary artery blood flow occurs predominantly during diastole.
  B. The left main stem artery divides into the left anterior descending and circumflex arteries.
  C. The circumflex artery supplies the majority of the interventricular septum.
  D. A myocardial infarct in the territory of the right coronary artery produces Q waves in leads V1 to V3.
  E. Myocardial infarction in the territory of the left anterior descending artery produces Q waves in the inferior chest leads on ECG.
  F. Occlusion of the circumflex artery may produce a tall R wave in lead V1 of the ECG.

102. Coronary artery surgery:

  A. Is more effective than medical therapy in returning patients to employment.
  B. Improves survival in isolated right coronary artery disease.
  C. Improves survival in left main stem disease.
  D. In uncomplicated cases has an operative mortality of 10–12%.
  E. Only 60% of vein grafts are patent at 10 years.
  F. Is no better in terms of survival than medical therapy in patients with triple vessel disease and poor left ventricular function.

(Answers overleaf)

100. A.   True.   It is three times as common.
   B.   True.
   C.   False.   Almost always distal to the left subclavian artery.
   D.   False.   Early correction leads to better results.
   E.   True.   As a result of left subclavian involvement.
   F.   True.

101. A.   True.   Intramyocardial vessels are compressed during systole.
   B.   True.
   C.   False.   The LAD and its septal vessels supply two-thirds, the right coronary up to one-third.
   D.   False.   Produces inferior changes (leads II, III and aVF).
   E.   False.   Produces changes in the anterior (V) leads.
   F.   True.   A true posterior infarct.

102. A.   False.   In purely 'economic' terms CABG is disappointing.
   B.   False.   Survival is good with medical treatment alone.
   C.   True.   The left main stem artery supplies a very large territory.
   D.   False.   Mortality is less than 1%.
   E.   True.   Internal mammary grafts have a better patency rate.
   F.   False.   Survival is improved by surgery — probably due to better left ventricular performance.

103 **The following therapies improve long-term survival in acute myocardial infarction:**
   A. Tissue plasminogen activator.
   B. Streptokinase given 36 hours after the onset of pain.
   C. Aspirin.
   D. Nifedipine.
   E. Atenolol.
   F. Immediate percutaneous transluminal angioplasty.

104. **The following cause a restrictive cardiomyopathy:**
   A. Alcohol.
   B. Sarcoidosis.
   C. Adriamycin.
   D. Cobalt.
   E. Endomyocardial fibrosis.
   F. Löffler's syndrome.

105. **Infective endocarditis:**
   A. Can occur on previously normal heart valves.
   B. Can be caused only by bacteria.
   C. *Streptococcus faecalis* is the commonest pathogen.
   D. Most commonly affects the mitral valve.
   E. Oral ampicillin (250 mg) 1 hour before dental manipulation and prescribed for 1 week thereafter is adequate prophylaxis.
   F. Can prolong the PR interval.

106. **The following statements of pericardial constriction are true:**
   A. Patients may present with ascites.
   B. The jugular venous pressure is often normal.
   C. The arterial pressure falls on inspiration.
   D. Echocardiography readily distinguishes this condition from a constrictive cardiomyopathy.
   E. Right-sided diastolic pressures greatly exceed left-sided ones.
   F. In chronic constriction due to infection with *Mycobacterium tuberculosis*, the cardiac symptoms will respond to antituberculous therapy.

(Answers overleaf)

103.
  A. **True.** This is a thrombolytic agent.
  B. **False.** No benefit has been shown at more than 24 hours. Maximum benefit occurs within the first few hours.
  C. **True.** As shown in the ISIS II trial.
  D. **False.**
  E. **True.** As shown in ISIS I.
  F. **False.** There is an appreciable immediate mortality from the procedure in these unstable patients.

104.
  A. **False.** Causes a dilated cardiomyopathy.
  B. **True.** Produces a granulomatous infiltration of the myocardium.
  C. **False.** Causes a dilated cardiomyopathy.
  D. **False.** Causes a dilated cardiomyopathy.
  E. **True.**
  F. **True.** Produces an eosinophilic infiltrate.

105.
  A. **True.** For example, in intravenous drug addicts or following severe staphylococcal sepsis.
  B. **False.** Fungal and rickettsial infections also occur.
  C. **False.** *Streptococcus viridans* is the most common pathogen on non-prosthetic valves.
  D. **True.** The valves are affected in order of mechanical loading.
  E. **False.** Amoxycillin (3 g) given 1 hour before the procedure is recommended for low-risk individuals.
  F. **True.** This indicates an aortic root abscess.

106.
  A. **True.** Symptoms of right heart failure are common.
  B. **False.** Invariably raised.
  C. **True.** 'Pulsus paradoxus' caused by the marked fall in stroke volume.
  D. **False.** The conditions are very difficult to distinguish.
  E. **False.** Equalisation of right and left ventricular end diastolic pressures is usual.
  F. **False.** The pericardium is usually calcified and requires operative treatment. The acute pericarditis may respond to antituberculous drugs and steroids.

107. In the treatment of hypertension:

A. Beta-blockers are included as first-line agents.

B. Angiotensin-converting enzyme inhibitors are the treatment of choice in renovascular hypertension.

C. Patients with a sustained diastolic pressure of over 90 mmHg require drug treatment.

D. Methyldopa should be avoided in pregnancy.

E. Beta-blockers are usually effective as sole agents in phaeochromocytoma.

F. Thiazide diuretics are useful in Conn's syndrome.

108. Aortic dissection:

A. May produce an early diastolic murmur best heard at the right sternal edge.

B. Should all be managed surgically following medical stabilisation.

C. Can be diagnosed by CT scanning.

D. Can be diagnosed by trans-oesophageal echocardiography.

E. May present with ECG changes suggesting an acute myocardial infarction.

F. Are divided into types A and B depending on the involvement of the descending aorta.

(Answers overleaf)

107. A. True. These are effective, although side-effects are common.
   B. False. This may lead to renal failure caused by loss of efferent glomerular arteriolar tone.
   C. False. A pressure of 100 mmHg or above is the present guideline, although debate continues.
   D. False. Trials have shown this to be a safe agent.
   E. False. An alpha-blocker is also required.
   F. False. A potassium-sparing diuretic is needed.

108. A. True. In type A dissections aortic regurgitation can occur.
   B. False. Type B dissections can be managed medically.
   C. True. Usually accurate, although angiography may be necessary.
   D. True. This technique may become the definitive non-invasive method.
   E. True. The coronary arteries may be involved in the dissection.
   F. False. They are separated depending on the involvement of the proximal ascending aorta.

15. Respiratory disease

109. In the normal respiratory system:

A. Total ventilation = alveolar ventilation – dead space ventilation.

B. Vital capacity + residual volume = total lung capacity.

C. A rise in $Paco_2$ causes a rise in pH.

D. The transfer factor is usually measured with CO.

E. Pulmonary blood flow is greater at the bases.

F. Haemoglobin is more than 90% saturated at a $PaO_2 > 8$ kPa (60 mmHg).

110. Lung function testing:

A. Shows a fall in residual volume in airflow obstruction.

B. Shows a restrictive defect in severe kyphoscoliosis.

C. Following pneumonectomy will show a normal KCO if the remaining lung is normal.

D. Compliance is increased in emphysema.

E. Shows a relatively greater fall in PEFR compared to FEV_1 in upper airway obstruction.

F. Shows a decreased gas transfer factor in lung haemorrhage.

111. In the interpretation of arterial blood gases:

A. Arterial oxygen content is partially determined by haemoglobin concentration.

B. Ventilation/perfusion mismatching is the commonest cause of hypoxia.

C. Central cyanosis occurs at oxygen saturations of less than 92%.

D. Acute hyperventilation increases pH.

E. $Paco_2$ is proportional to alveolar ventilation.

F. Blood HCO_3 falls in patients with chronic CO_2 retention.

(Answers overleaf)

109. A. False. Total ventilation = alveolar ventilation (V_A) + dead space ventilation (V_D).

  B. True.

  C. False. Acute hypercapnia produces a respiratory acidosis with a fall in pH.

  D. True.

  E. True. Caused by gravity.

  F. True.

110. A. False. Gas trapping increases the residual volume.

  B. True. May lead to respiratory failure in some patients.

  C. True. The KCO is the transfer factor corrected for alveolar volume and is therefore normal providing the remaining lung is normal.

  D. True. A result of the destruction of elastic support.

  E. True. Best seen in the 'flattened' profile of the flow volume loop.

  F. False. More CO is bound to the free haemoglobin and gas transfer rises.

111. A. True. A product of the oxygen-combining capacity of haemoglobin, haemoglobin concentration, and oxygen saturation.

  B. True.

  C. False. Cyanosis usually occurs only at oxygen saturations below 85%.

  D. True. $Paco_2$ falls, leading to a respiratory alkalosis.

  E. False. Inversely proportional to alveolar ventilation.

  F. False. There is a compensatory rise in bicarbonate retained by the kidney.

112. The following symptoms occur in chest disease:

A. Cough can be a presenting feature in achalasia of the cardia.

B. Sputum production is unusual in alveolar cell carcinoma.

C. Life-threatening haemoptysis occurs in bronchiectasis.

D. Significant tracheal stenosis can cause a predominantly expiratory wheeze.

E. Clubbing can occur in mesothelioma.

F. Hypertrophic pulmonary osteoarthropathy is most commonly associated with oat cell carcinoma of the lung.

113. In the radiology of the chest:

A. The right hilum is below the left hilum.

B. An air bronchogram indicates the presence of patent, air-filled bronchi.

C. Kerley B lines are produced by distended lymphatics.

D. The horizontal fissure lies between the right upper and lower lobe.

E. Computerised tomographic scanning is poor at imaging the mediastinum.

F. Collapse of the middle lobe obscures the right hemidiaphragm.

114. In acute pneumonia:

A. *Streptococcus* pneumonia is usually hospital acquired.

B. *Haemophilus influenzae* is the commonest infection in patients with chronic bronchitis and emphysema.

C. Staphylococcal pneumonia characteristically follows viral influenza.

D. High-dose amoxycillin is usually an effective treatment in *Legionella* pneumonia.

E. *Mycoplasma* pneumonia often produces a neutrophil leucocytosis.

F. The risk of contracting Q fever pneumonia is increased in sewage workers.

(Answers overleaf)

112. **A.** **True.** Due to recurrent aspiration.
  B. **False.** Some patients produce large volumes of sputum.
  C. **True.** Other common causes of severe haemoptysis are cavitating tuberculosis and lung carcinoma.
  D. **False.** The wheeze is characteristically inspiratory.
  E. **True.**
  F. **False.** Most commonly associated with squamous cell carcinoma.

113. **A.** **True.**
  B. **True.** This sign can exclude a proximal obstruction (usually a tumour) in a densely opacified lung field.
  C. **True.**
  D. **False.** The horizontal fissure lies between the upper and middle lobes.
  E. **False.** This is often the investigation of choice.
  F. **False.** It obscures the right heart border; an example of the 'silhouette' sign.

114. **A.** **False.** It is the commonest cause of community acquired pneumonia.
  B. **True.**
  C. **True.**
  D. **False.** The disease is sensitive to erythromycin, ciprofloxacin and rifampicin.
  E. **False.** In *Mycoplasma* and other viral-like pneumonias the neutrophil count is usually normal.
  F. **False.** It is usually contracted from animals and sheep. Vets and slaughterhouse workers are occupational groups at risk.

115. In immunocompromised patients with pneumonia:

A. The plain chest radiograph usually distinguishes leukaemic infiltration from pneumonia.

B. Bronchoscopy is hazardous and should be avoided.

C. Focal changes on the plain radiograph favour a bacterial origin for the pneumonia.

D. Cytomegalovirus infection is the commonest cause of diffuse chest radiograph abnormality in HIV-positive patients.

E. Steroid therapy is contraindicated in severe *Pneumocystis* pneumonia.

F. *Nocardia* pneumonia characteristically cavitates.

116. The following statements regarding pulmonary infection with *Mycobacterium tuberculosis* are correct:

A. Twelve months of drug therapy is standard.

B. Single-agent drug therapy is often effective in uncomplicated cases.

C. Rifampicin can produce optic neuritis.

D. Streptomycin is a first-line antituberculous drug.

E. Post-primary tuberculosis commonly affects the upper lobes of the lung.

F. Rifampicin is used as prophylaxis is against *M. tuberculosis* infection in HIV-positive patients.

117. In patients with bronchiectasis the following features suggest a specific aetiology:

A. Finger clubbing.

B. Small-bowel obstruction.

C. Massive haemoptysis.

D. Peripheral oedema.

E. Dextrocardia.

F. Blood eosinophilia.

118. Cystic fibrosis:

A. Is inherited in an autosomal dominant manner.

B. Increases the sodium content of sweat.

C. Can cause malabsorption.

D. Causes diabetes insipidus.

E. Typically causes recurrent *Klebsiella* chest infections.

F. Increases total lung capacity.

(Answers overleaf)

115. A. False. The conditions are often radiologically indistinguishable.
    B. False. Except in the most critically ill patients this is a safe and well tolerated procedure with a high diagnostic yield.
    C. True. Diffuse changes suggest an opportunistic infection.
    D. False. *Pneumocystis* pneumonia is the commonest cause.
    E. False. Clinical trials have now demonstrated increased survival if steroids are given early.
    F. True.

116. A. False. Six-month regimens have now been shown to be highly effective.
    B. False. Combination chemotherapy is essential to prevent the emergence of drug-resistant organisms.
    C. False. Ethambutol is associated with this complication.
    D. False. Rifampicin, isoniazid, pyrazinamide and ethambutol are the first-line agents in economically developed countries.
    E. True.
    F. True. Isoniazid is the agent used.

117. A. False. Common in all forms of severe disease.
    B. True. Meconium ileus equivalent in cystic fibrosis.
    C. False. Occurs in any form.
    D. False. Fluid overload due to cor pulmonale occurs in all forms of advanced disease.
    E. True. Kartagener's syndrome (ciliary dysfunction).
    F. True. Allergic bronchopulmonary aspergillosis.

118. A. False. Autosomal recessive.
    B. True. The cellular deficit is probably in chloride transport.
    C. True. Due to pancreatic insufficiency.
    D. False. Diabetes mellitus is relatively common.
    E. False. *Pseudomonas* and staphylococcal pneumonia are common.
    F. True. Airflow obstruction is common leading to gas trapping.

119. In asthma:
A. PEFR is highest in the mornings.
B. The residual volume is often increased.
C. High oxygen concentrations can be safely given in severe attacks.
D. Pulsus paradoxus is a poor guide to severity.
E. Calcium antagonists are safe antihypertensive drugs.
F. The transfer factor is often low.

120. In the treatment of acute, severe asthma:
A. Sedatives may be needed in agitated patients.
B. High concentrations of oxygen should be given before arterial blood gases are available.
C. Intravenous theophylline should be given immediately.
D. Nebulised β_2 agonists are ineffective.
E. A raised Paco$_2$ indicates the need for immediate mechanical ventilation.
F. In pregnancy, oral steroids are contraindicated.

121. In chronic bronchitis and emphysema:
A. The FEV$_1$/FVC ratio is usually reduced.
B. Gas transfer is often normal in advanced emphysema.
C. Domiciliary oxygen therapy prolongs survival in patients with advanced disease.
D. Cessation of smoking has no impact on the rate of decline of lung function in COAD.
E. The five-year survival of patients with cor pulmonale is approximately 30%.
F. Emphysematous changes occurring predominantly in the lower zones suggest α_1-antitrypsin deficiency.

122. In the sleep apnoeas:
A. Systemic hypertension is common.
B. Morning headaches can be a presenting feature.
C. Anaemia is common in advanced disease.
D. Weight loss is an effective treatment in the central type.
E. Protriptyline may be an effective treatment.
F. Most patients are asymptomatic during the daytime.

(Answers overleaf)

119. **A. False.**   PEFR is lowest in the mornings ('morning dipping'). This is the characteristic diurnal variation in PEFR.
    B. True.   Due to gas trapping with airflow obstruction.
    C. True.   Ventilatory control is normal and a rising $Paco_2$ indicates very severe disease and the need for more intensive therapy.
    D. False.   There is a good correlation between the degree of paradox and the severity of the attack.
    E. True.   Beta-blockers are contraindicated.
    F. False.   The transfer factor is usually normal or even raised. Low TLCO suggests the presence of emphysema.

120. **A. False.**   Agitation often indicates that the patient is hypoxic, frightened, and close to exhaustion.
    B. True.   Unlike patients with chronic bronchitis, CO_2 narcosis will not be precipitated.
    C. False.   The patient may already be taking theophylline.
    D. False.   Provided the patient can cooperate with the treatment.
    E. False.   A significant number will have mildly raised $Paco_2$ initially which should fall with treatment. A $Paco_2$ that rises despite treatment indicates the need for ventilation.
    F. False.   Fetal mortality is increased in pregnant asthmatics with poorly controlled asthma.

121. **A. True.**   Airflow obstruction is invariably present.
    B. False.   Reduced due to loss of lung vasculature.
    C. True.   As shown in the Medical Research Council and National Institutes of Health clinical trials.
    D. False.   There is good evidence that the rate of decline decreases.
    E. True.   Domiciliary oxygen therapy improves survival to approximately 45%.
    F. True.   Probably related to increased basal blood flow.

122. **A. True.**
    B. True.   Due to CO_2 retention overnight.
    C. False.   Polycythaemia is common.
    D. False.   Weight loss is effective in the obstructive variety.
    E. True.   The drug reduces REM sleep during which the apnoeas occur.
    F. False.   Gradual intellectual deterioration and daytime sleepiness are common.

123. In respiratory failure:

A. The Pao_2 is by definition less than 10 kPa.

B. Obstructive sleep apnoea is a recognised cause.

C. A widened alveolar–arterial gradient indicates intrinsic lung disease.

D. The $Paco_2$ is often normal in a spontaneously breathing myasthenic patient with respiratory failure.

E. Oxygen therapy should always be commenced with an FIO_2 of 24%.

F. The arterial–mixed venous oxygen content difference is a useful index of tissue oxygenation.

124. In pulmonary thromboembolic disease:

A. The ECG is often diagnostic.

B. Approximately 70% of patients with a pulmonary embolus will have deep-vein thrombosis on venography.

C. Streptokinase is no longer a recommended treatment.

D. Most patients should receive anticoagulation for at least 1 year.

E. In pregnancy, warfarin should be used for treatment.

F. A normal ventilation/perfusion scan will exclude pulmonary emboli in most cases.

125. In sarcoidosis:

A. Serum angiotension levels are often reduced.

B. The eye is involved in over 90% of cases.

C. If bilateral hilar lymphadenopathy occurs alone then complete resolution will occur in the majority of cases.

D. Hypocalcaemia can be a presenting feature.

E. Diabetes insipidus can occur.

F. A predominantly neutrophil leucocytosis occurs in broncho-alveolar lavage fluid.

126. The following multisystem diseases and lung diseases go together:

A. Systemic sclerosis and lung nodules.

B. Rheumatoid arthritis and pleural effusions.

C. Systemic sclerosis and pulmonary fibrosis.

D. Wegener's granulomatosis and fibrosing alveolitis.

E. Churg–Strauss syndrome and asthma.

F. Systemic lupus erythematosus and pulmonary hypertension.

(Answers overleaf)

123 A. False. Defined as a Pao$_2$ of less than 8 kPa.
  B. True. Patients with advanced disease can present with unexplained hypoxia, hypercapnia and cor pulmonale.
  C. True. The A–a gradient is widened by venous admixture (true shunt or V/Q mismatch).
  D. False. Raised. Neuromuscular disease produces alveolar hypoventilation, and Paco$_2$ therefore rises.
  E. False. Only patients at risk of CO_2 retention should be started on low FIO$_2$.
  F. True. If oxygen delivery is inadequate, the arterial–mixed venous oxygen content difference widens.

124. A. False. The ECG is often normal or non-specifically abnormal. The classic SI, QIII, TIII changes are rarely seen.
  B. True. This may be useful in determining the likelihood of a pulmonary embolus.
  C. False. Streptokinase should be used in massive emboli.
  D. False. Three to six months in uncomplicated cases is adequate.
  E. False. Warfarin is teratogenic. Subcutaneous heparin is the agent of choice.
  F. True. An abnormal scan is, however, non-specific in some cases.

125. A. False. Levels are often increased.
  B. False. Eye involvement occurs in less than 25% of cases.
  C. True.
  D. False. Hypercalcaemia occurs due to increased calcium absorption from the gut.
  E. True. Involvement of the hypothalamus and posterior pituitary is uncommon but well recognised.
  F. False. A predominantly lymphocytic fluid is seen.

126. A. False. Nodules are a feature of rheumatoid lung.
  B. True. Up to 30% of patients will develop effusions at some stage in their illness.
  C. True. This is the most common form of lung involvement.
  D. False. Wegener's granulomatosis causes destructive lesions of the upper respiratory tract and pulmonary nodules that often cavitate.
  E. True.
  F. True. Associated with anticardiolipin antibodies and pulmonary thrombosis.

127. Exposure to dust causes the following lung problems:

A. In coal miners' pneumoconiosis; large, irregular upper-lobe masses are likely to be caused by adenocarcinoma.

B. Asbestosis can cause finger clubbing.

C. The pleural plagues associated with asbestos exposure are usually benign.

D. Finger clubbing is uncommon in extrinsic allergic alveolitis.

E. Hilar calcification occurs in berylliosis.

F. Extrinsic allergic alveolitis causes predominantly basal fibrosis.

128. In the adult respiratory distress syndrome (ARDS):

A. The pulmonary artery wedge pressure is characteristically elevated.

B. The pulmonary endothelium is damaged early in the course of the illness.

C. Lung compliance is increased.

D. The use of positive end expiratory pressure increases compliance.

E. The mortality exceeds 40% despite modern treatment.

F. Mortality is decreased by the early use of high-dose steroids.

129. In carcinoma of the bronchus:

A. Squamous cell carcinoma is the commonest form.

B. Ectopic ACTH production is commonest with squamous cell tumours.

C. The 5-year survival following surgery for lung cancer is approximately 70%.

D. The median survival in untreated small-cell lung cancer is about 4 months.

E. Hypertrophic pulmonary osteoarthropathy (HPOA) is most commonly associated with squamous cell carcinoma.

F. Radiotherapy significantly prolongs survival in lung cancer.

(Answers overleaf)

127. A. **False.** Characteristic of progressive massive fibrosis. This can resemble carcinoma radiologically.
    B. **True.**
    C. **True.** To be differentiated from mesothelioma.
    D. **True.** In marked contrast to cryptogenic fibrosing alveolitis.
    E. **False.** This is seen in silicosis, the so-called 'egg-shell calcification'.
    F. **False.** It produces predominantly upper-zone fibrosis.

128. A. **False.** A raised wedge pressure suggests cardiogenic pulmonary oedema.
    B. **True.** This is the cause of the low-pressure permeability oedema which characterises the condition.
    C. **False.** Lung compliance is reduced. The lung becomes 'stiff'.
    D. **True.** Compliance improves because functional residual capacity is increased, thereby altering the point on the pressure–volume curve that the lung is operating upon.
    E. **True.** The mortality has remained between 50 and 70% since the syndrome was first described 20 years ago.
    F. **False.** Two multicentre controlled trials showed no benefit. Mortality may increase in septic patients with ARDS given steroids.

129. A. **True.** Small cell (oat cell) carcinoma is the next most frequent.
    B. **False.** It is commonest with oat cell carcinoma. Hypercalcaemia is most common with squamous cell tumours.
    C. **False.** Approximately 25% of patients survive 5 years.
    D. **True.** Chemotherapy can prolong median survival to approximately 1 year.
    E. **True.**
    F. **False.** In general, radiotherapy is useful only in symptom palliation.

130. The following are features of unusual thoracic tumours:

A. Mediastinal teratomas usually arise in the posterior mediastinum.

B. Mediastinal thymomas usually arise in the anterior mediastinum.

C. Thymomas are associated with multiple sclerosis.

D. Malignant mesotheliomas rarely produce thoracic pain.

E. Alveolar cell cancer is more common in cigarette smokers.

F. Less than 10% of patients with lung carcinoid tumours present with the carcinoid syndrome.

131. The following conditions typically cause a pleural effusion in which the fluid is a transudate:

A. Pulmonary infarction.

B. Hypothyroidism.

C. Rheumatoid arthritis.

D. Constrictive pericarditis.

E. Cardiac failure.

F. Meigs' syndrome.

132. Spontaneous pneumothorax:

A. Is commoner in females than males.

B. May present with a cough.

C. May be associated with Marfan's syndrome.

D. Has a relapse rate of about 20%.

E. May be associated with menstruation.

F. Seldom produces symptoms in patients with cystic fibrosis.

(Answers overleaf)

130. A. **False.** Anterior mediastinum.
     B. **True.**
     C. **False.** They are associated with myasthenia gravis.
     D. **False.** Severe chest wall pain is a common presenting feature.
     E. **False.**
     F. **True.** Many present with signs and symptoms of endobronchial obstruction.

131. A. **False.** The effusion is an exudate.
     B. **True.**
     C. **False.** Typically, the fluid is an exudate.
     D. **True.**
     E. **True.**
     F. **True.**

132. A. **False.** Commoner in males.
     B. **True.**
     C. **True.**
     D. **True.**
     E. **True.** This is a catamenial pneumothorax.
     F. **False.** Even a small pneumothorax may cause severe breathlessness in patients with pre-existing lung disease.

16. Critical care medicine

133. In critically ill patients with cardiovascular problems:

A. Central venous pressure reflects left ventricular filling pressures.

B. Thermodilution right ventricular cardiac output can be measured by the injection of cold saline into the proximal pulmonary artery.

C. The cardiac index is the cardiac output normalised for body weight.

D. Urinary osmolarity is high in hypovolaemic shock.

E. Raised lactate levels indicate a decompensating circulation.

F. Measurement of the cardiac index can distinguish hypovolaemic from cardiogenic shock.

134. In septic shock and multisystem organ failure:

A. Hypotension is often caused by a decrease in peripheral vascular resistance.

B. Fever is invariable.

C. Vasoconstrictor agents are contraindicated.

D. Mixed venous oxygen tensions can be inappropriately high.

E. If three or more organ systems fail the mortality is 25%.

F. Vascular endothelial damage is a common feature.

135. In patients being mechanically ventilated:

A. $Paco_2$ does not reflect the adequacy of alveolar ventilation.

B. Positive end expiratory pressure may reduce the cardiac index (CI).

C. Hyperphosphataemia may impair respiratory muscle contractility.

D. Most patients with a spontaneous vital capacity of 5 ml/kg will successfully wean from mechanical ventilation.

E. Calorie requirements are typically low in patients with severe burns.

F. Gastric motility is increased by erythromycin.

(Answers overleaf)

133. A. **False.** It reflects right ventricular filling. In critically ill patients this may poorly reflect left ventricular filling.

    B. **False.** The injection is made proximally in the right atrium and the temperature is recorded by thermistor in the pulmonary artery.

    C. **False.** The index corrects for body surface area.

    D. **True.**

    E. **True.**

    F. **False.** Cardiac index falls in both conditions. Measurement of pulmonary artery wedge pressure distinguishes between these two conditions.

134. A. **True.** The cardiac output is often normal or elevated early in the course of sepsis.

    B. **False.** Hypothermia is well recognised in the early stages.

    C. **False.** Constrictor agents may be useful in intractable hypotension.

    D. **True.** This is caused by an inability of the peripheral tissues to utilise oxygen.

    E. **False.** Mortality is greater than 90%.

    F. **True.** This is likely to be the common pathological feature in septic shock syndromes.

135. A. **False.** $Paco_2$ still reflects the adequacy of CO_2 clearance and therefore alveolar ventilation.

    B. **True.** By decreasing cardiac output:
O_2 delivery = cardiac output × arterial O_2 content.

    C. **True.**

    D. **False.** In general, more than 20 ml/kg is needed.

    E. **False.** Calorie requirements may be 100% higher.

    F. **True.** And also by metoclopramide.

136. In critically ill patients with head injuries:

   A. Hypocapnia reduces cerebral blood flow.
   B. Severe hypoxaemia (Pao_2 < 5 kPa) reduces cerebral blood flow.
   C. Mean cerebral artery perfusion pressure = mean arterial pressure – mean intracranial pressure.
   D. Intermittent positive pressure ventilation reduces intracranial pressure by reducing venous drainage.
   E. Paralysing drugs should be used to prevent intractable convulsions.
   F. The mortality is greater than 50% in patients with a Glasgow Coma Scale of 12 or greater.

(Answers overleaf)

136. A. True. This is the rationale for controlled hyperventilation.
B. False. Severe hypoxia increases cerebral blood flow.
C. True. Hence the need to control intracranial pressure.
D. False. This can increase intracranial pressure by this mechanism as the pressure is transmitted retrogradely.
E. False. This will only mask the motor features of the convulsion.
F. False. Low scores are associated with a high mortality.

17. Gastrointestinal disease

137. In the investigation of gastrointestinal disease:

A. The Schilling test may be used to distinguish between B_{12} deficiency following ileal resection and that occurring secondary to a blind loop.

B. A barium swallow should be performed prior to endoscopy in a patient presenting with dysphagia.

C. A breath hydrogen test may be used to assess small intestinal transit.

D. Reduced gastric acid secretory response to pentagastrin is common in duodenal ulcer.

E. Insulin hypoglycaemia reduces gastric acid secretion via the vagus.

F. Small intestinal permeability to lactulose is increased in untreated coeliac disease.

138. The following are true of gut regulatory peptides:

A. Secretin stimulates pancreatic bicarbonate secretion.

B. Gastrin levels are reduced in Zollinger–Ellison syndrome.

C. Gastrin is produced in the gastric antrum.

D. Meal-stimulated plasma cholecystokinin levels are raised in untreated coeliac disease.

E. Somatostatin reduces intestinal secretions.

F. Enteroglucagon increases gastric emptying.

139. The following are recognised causes of oral ulceration:

A. Ulcerative colitis.

B. Coeliac disease.

C. Sulphonamide treatment.

D. Phenytoin treatment.

E. Lichen planus.

F. Coxsackie B viruses.

(Answers overleaf)

137. **A.** **False.** Both lead to malabsorption of B_{12}–intrinsic factor complex.
   B. **True.** To avoid risk of perforation at endoscopy.
   C. **True.** After administration of a carbohydrate test meal.
   D. **False.** There is increased response to pentagastrin.
   E. **False.** It stimulates acid secretion via the vagus; it can be used to assess efficacy of surgical vagotomy.
   F. **True.**

138. **A.** **True.** Released from the duodenum.
   B. **False.** They are raised due to release from gastrinoma.
   C. **True.**
   D. **False.** They are reduced.
   E. **True.** It is released from the pancreas and the gut.
   F. **False.** Delays gastric emptying.

139. **A.** **False.** Crohn's disease is.
   B. **True.** It may be the presenting feature.
   C. **True.** In association with erythema multiforme.
   D. **False.** It causes gum hypertrophy.
   E. **True.** However, it more commonly causes hyperkeratotic plaques.
   F. **False.** Coxsackie A causes both herpangina and hand, foot and mouth disease.

140. The following are true of oesophageal carcinoma:

A. The majority arise in the upper third.

B. Adenocarcinoma is the most common type.

C. The incidence is increased in coeliac disease.

D. Dysphagia for liquids is an early symptom.

E. Five-year survival after radical surgery is around 50%.

F. The incidence is higher in females than males over the age of 60.

141. In a patient with acute gastrointestinal bleeding:

A. The passage of melaena implies bleeding from above the ileocaecal junction.

B. The passage of fresh blood per rectum may be due to a bleeding duodenal ulcer.

C. Blood should be given only if the haemoglobin is less than 10 g/dl.

D. Early surgery should be avoided if the patient is over 60 years of age.

E. A Mallory–Weiss tear, if this is the cause, is usually visible at endoscopy.

F. Haemorrhage from oesophageal varices may be controlled by an infusion of desmopressin.

142. In peptic ulceration:

A. Duodenal ulcers are four times as common as gastric ulcers.

B. Duodenogastric reflux is important in the pathogenesis of duodenal ulcer.

C. A family history is uncommon in gastric ulcer.

D. Duodenal ulcers are associated with blood group A.

E. Sucralfate acts by reducing gastric acid production.

F. Infection with *Campylobacter jejuni* may be a predisposing factor.

143. In coeliac disease:

A. Presentation in adolescence is unusual.

B. Constipation may be a presenting feature.

C. Hypersplenism is common.

D. Products made with rye flour are safe.

E. There is an association with HLA-B27 tissue type.

F. The rash of associated dermatitis herpetiformis affects predominantly extensor surfaces.

(Answers overleaf)

140. A. False. Only 15% arise in the upper third; 40% arise in the middle third, and 45% in the lower third.
   B. False. The majority are squamous cell carcinomas.
   C. True. Also increased in smokers, alcoholics and achalasia.
   D. False. Initially for solids.
   E. False. Five year survival is 30% or less.
   F. False. It is higher in males.

141. A. False. It may occur with proximal colonic lesions.
   B. True. This occurs only if there is brisk bleeding and rapid intestinal transit.
   C. False. Blood should be given if there are signs of shock.
   D. False. Mortality is greatest in this age group if bleeding persists.
   E. True.
   F. False. A vasopressin infusion is used; it reduces portal vein pressure by vasoconstriction of the splanchnic bed.

142. A. True.
   B. False. Reflux of alkaline juice through the pylorus may be important in gastric ulcer.
   C. True. However, it is common in duodenal ulcer.
   D. False. They are associated with blood group O.
   E. False. It is a mucosal protectant.
   F. False. Infection with *Helicobacter pylori* is a predisposing factor.

143. A. True. It is more common in early childhood and in the third and fourth decades.
   B. True. However, diarrhoea is much more common.
   C. False. Hyposplenism is present in most patients.
   D. False. Patients must avoid wheat, rye, barley and, possibly, oats.
   E. False. The association is with the HLA-B8-DR3 tissue type.
   F. True.

144. The following are recognised causes of secretory diarrhoea:
  A. Cholera.
  B. Thyrotoxicosis.
  C. Laxative abuse.
  D. Ulcerative colitis.
  E. Medullary carcinoma of the thyroid.
  F. Hypolactasia.

145. The following are recognised causes of constipation:
  A. Antacids containing aluminium salts.
  B. Ulcerative proctitis.
  C. Iron therapy.
  D. Hypocalcaemia.
  E. Lead poisoning.
  F. Hypokalaemia.

146. The following are true of carcinoma of the colon:
  A. There is an equal sex incidence.
  B. The transverse colon is the most common site.
  C. Genetic factors may be involved in the aetiology.
  D. Distant metastases are present with a Dukes' C tumour.
  E. The incidence in Japan is lower than in Western countries.
  F. Adjuvant chemotherapy improves the prognosis of operable tumours.

147. The following features favour the diagnosis of Crohn's disease rather than ulcerative colitis:
  A. Transmural inflammation of the bowel wall.
  B. Passage of blood and mucus per rectum.
  C. Pyoderma gangrenosum.
  D. Response to treatment with sulphasalazine.
  E. Oxalate renal stones.
  F. Onset in early adult life.

(Answers overleaf)

144. **A.** **True.** Due to the action of an enterotoxin.
    B. **False.** Diarrhoea in this case is due to rapid small intestinal transit.
    C. **True.** Especially phenolphthalein.
    D. **False.** This condition is associated with inflammatory diarrhoea.
    E. **True.** Hormonal.
    F. **False.** Osmotic diarrhoea due to failure of lactose digestion.

145. **A.** **True.** However, magnesium salts can cause diarrhoea.
    B. **True.** Constipation proximal to inflamed rectum.
    C. **True.**
    D. **False.** Hypercalcaemia is a recognised cause.
    E. **True.**
    F. **True.**

146. **A.** **True.** However, carcinoma of the rectum is more common in males.
    B. **False.** The rectum, sigmoid and right side of colon are the commonest sites.
    C. **True.** The incidence is greatly increased in familial polyposis coli.
    D. **False.** There is spread to local lymph nodes only; distant metastases occur in Dukes' D tumours.
    E. **True.** Factors associated with Western lifestyle increase the incidence.
    F. **True.** Postoperative chemotherapy improves the prognosis in Dukes' B and more advanced tumours.

147. **A.** **True.** Ulcerative colitis primarily involves the mucosa.
    B. **False.** This occurs in both Crohn's disease and ulcerative colitis.
    C. **False.** This occurs in both conditions.
    D. **False.** The response is better in ulcerative colitis.
    E. **True.** Increased colonic bile acids in terminal ileal disease enhance oxalate absorption.
    F. **False.** This is the most common time for both conditions to present.

148. **The following are recognised non-intestinal manifestations of inflammatory bowel disease:**
    A. Erythema marginatum.
    B. Episcleritis.
    C. Pericarditis.
    D. Sacro-iliitis.
    E. Amyloid.
    F. Cholangiocarcinoma.

149. **In ulcerative colitis:**
    A. Anaemia, if present, is usually macrocytic.
    B. Histology of the affected bowel shows mucosal granulomas.
    C. Corticosteroids are the mainstay of treatment of the severe acute attack.
    D. Most patients improve during pregnancy.
    E. The incidence of carcinoma is not increased if the disease is confined to the rectum.
    F. Less than 10% of patients will require colectomy.

150. **The following are characteristic features of functional bowel disorders:**
    A. Onset of symptoms in the fifth decade.
    B. Tendency to run in families.
    C. Passage of mucus in stool.
    D. Weight loss.
    E. Increased daily stool weight.
    F. Exaggerated sinus arrhythmia.

(Answers overleaf)

148. **A. False.** However, erythema nodosum is; erythema marginatum occurs in rheumatic fever.
   B. True. Conjunctivitis and uveitis are also manifestations.
   C. False.
   D. True.
   E. True. This is so in Crohn's disease; it may also occur within the gastrointestinal tract.
   F. True.

149. **A. False.** It is hypochromic, microcytic, due to blood loss.
   B. False. Granulomas are a feature of Crohn's disease, not ulcerative colitis.
   C. True. Rectal and/or systemic.
   D. True.
   E. True. The risk is greatest in patients who have suffered from pancolitiis for over 10 years.
   F. False. Up to 25% of patients require colectomy within 5–10 years.

150. **A. False.** Onset occurs in the third and fourth decades; onset over the age of 40 is more suggestive of organic disease.
   B. True. However, there is no clear pattern of inheritance.
   C. True. However, not blood.
   D. False. This suggests organic disease.
   E. False. Stool weight is normal.
   F. True. Indicative of autonomic overactivity.

151. In chronic pancreatitis:

A. Pancreatic endocrine function usually fails early on.
B. Steatorrhoea results from cholecystokinin deficiency.
C. Gallstones are the most common underlying cause.
D. Serum amylase levels are usually normal.
E. The disease may be inherited as an autosomal dominant condition.
F. There may be an associated vitamin B_{12} deficiency.

152. Cystic fibrosis:

A. Is inherited as an autosomal recessive condition.
B. Is characterised by a low sweat sodium concentration.
C. Is almost always fatal before the age of 10.
D. Leads to steatorrhoea which responds poorly to pancreatic enzyme supplements.
E. May be complicated by cirrhosis of the liver.
F. In an affected fetus in utero, may lead to maternal oligohydramnios.

(Answers overleaf)

151. **A.** **False.** Exocrine function is lost relatively early; endocrine function fails only in advanced disease.
    B. **False.** It results from failure of lipase secretion in response to cholecystokinin.
    C. **False.** They are a common cause of acute pancreatitis, but only a rare cause of chronic pancreatitis.
    D. **True.** However, they are raised in acute pancreatitis.
    E. **True.** This is a rare hereditary form.
    F. **True.** The pancreas secretes a protease required for B_{12} absorption.

152. **A.** **True.**
    B. **False.** It is characterised by high sweat sodium and chloride.
    C. **False.** Many now survive into adulthood.
    D. **False.** There is a good response, especially if given with H_2-receptor antagonists.
    E. **True.**
    F. **False.** Maternal polyhydramnios occurs due to fetal meconium ileus.

18. Liver and biliary tract disease

153. In a patient with jaundice:
A. Generalised itching implies extrahepatic biliary obstruction.
B. The presence of leuconychia is suggestive of chronic liver disease.
C. Bilirubinuria suggests haemolysis.
D. Oral cholecystography is the best way of diagnosing gallstones.
E. A raised gamma-glutamyl transpeptidase is a less specific marker of cholestasis than a raised alkaline phosphatase.
F. Normal calibre intrahepatic bile ducts on ultrasound examination excludes extrahepatic obstruction.

154. In hepatitis B infection:
A. Transmission is usually by the faecal–oral route.
B. The incubation period is normally more than 4 weeks.
C. Chronic carriage occurs in only about 10% of neonatal infection.
D. The presence of hepatitis B 'e' antigen in the serum is a marker of infectivity.
E. Infection with Delta virus occurs only in chronic HBsAg carriers.
F. Antibodies to core proteins (anti-HBc) appear in the serum before antibodies to surface antigen (anti-HBs).

155. Fulminant hepatic failure:
A. Occurs commonly in severe aspirin poisoning.
B. May result from treatment with antituberculous drugs.
C. May be complicated by renal failure.
D. Should be treated by a high protein diet.
E. Is always accompanied by jaundice.
F. Usually leads to chronic liver disease in those who survive.

(Answers overleaf)

153. A. False. It occurs also in intrahepatic cholestasis.
    B. True. It reflects hypoalbuminaemia.
    C. False. Unconjugated bilirubin does not get into the urine.
    D. False. Ultrasound is better; oral cholecystography is no good if there is biliary obstruction.
    E. True. Gamma-glutamyl transpeptidase is also raised in hepatitis, and by alcohol.
    F. False. It can take several days for them to dilate.

154. A. False. Parenteral and sexual contact.
    B. True. A mean of 12 weeks.
    C. False. Approximately 90%.
    D. True. It implies active viral replication.
    E. False. It is possible to have acute coinfection with both hepatitis B and Delta viruses.
    F. True. Anti-HBc appears before onset of symptoms; anti-HBs appears as the virus is cleared.

155. A. False. It occurs in paracetamol poisoning.
    B. True. It may result from a rare complication of both isoniazid and rifampicin treatment.
    C. True. Due to endotoxaemia/septicaemia; the prognosis is poor.
    D. False. Encephalopathy is controlled by dietary protein restriction.
    E. False. Jaundice may be absent in rapidly progressive cases.
    F. False. Most who survive recover completely.

156. In gallstone disease:

A. Cholesterol stones are seen commonly in chronic haemolysis.

B. Most cholesterol stones are not visible on plain abdominal X-ray.

C. Stones in the common bile duct frequently cause cholangitis with Gram-positive bacteria.

D. Pigment stones are the commonest variety.

E. Empyema of the gallbladder is best treated conservatively with antibiotics.

F. There is a higher prevalence amongst elderly than middle-aged women.

157. In chronic alcoholic liver disease:

A. Reversible fatty change (steatosis) is commonly seen on liver biopsy.

B. Abstinence from alcohol does not improve the prognosis once cirrhosis has developed.

C. Steatosis progresses to cirrhosis in the majority of cases.

D. A raised mean corpuscular volume suggests continuing alcohol consumption.

E. The progression is faster in individuals with the HLA-B8 histocompatibility antigen.

F. Mallory's hyaline (perinuclear eosinophilic inclusion bodies) is a pathognomonic histological feature.

158. Chronic active hepatitis:

A. May follow acute hepatitis A.

B. Is associated with raised serum levels of IgM in the autoimmune type.

C. Is characterised by piecemeal necrosis of periportal hepatocytes.

D. May be caused by methyldopa.

E. When due to chronic hepatitis B infection, is best treated with corticosteroids.

F. Should be treated with cyclophosphamide in combination with corticosteroids if of autoimmune aetiology.

(Answers overleaf)

156. A. False. Pigment stones are seen.
   B. True. Only about 10% are radio-opaque.
   C. False. Gram-negative bacteria are involved.
   D. False. Mixed cholesterol stones are commonest.
   E. False. Surgical or percutaneous drainage is required in addition.
   F. True. The prevalence rises with increasing age.

157. A. True. It is the most consistent finding.
   B. False. The prognosis is greatly improved by complete abstinence.
   C. False. Most cases do not progress.
   D. True. It is a marker of recent alcohol consumption.
   E. True. HLA-B8 is associated with organ-specific autoimmunity.
   F. False. It is seen also in Wilson's disease and in primary biliary cirrhosis.

158. A. False. It may follow hepatitis B, C and Delta virus infection.
   B. False. It is associated with raised IgG; IgM is raised in primary biliary cirrhosis.
   C. True. This is a characteristic histological feature.
   D. True. Drugs are an important cause.
   E. False. Steroids are of no benefit.
   F. False. Azathioprine is used in combination with steroids in hepatitis of the autoimmune type.

159. The following are features of primary biliary cirrhosis:
   A. 90% of cases occur in women.
   B. Anti-smooth muscle antibodies are usually detectable in the serum.
   C. Abdominal pain is a common symptom.
   D. Corticosteroids are the treatment of choice.
   E. The disease usually presents in the fifth or sixth decade.
   F. There is an association with the HLA-A3 tissue type.

160. In idiopathic haemochromatosis:
   A. Serum ferritin levels are low.
   B. The characteristic pigmentation is due to increased melanin in the skin.
   C. There is usually an underlying haemolytic anaemia.
   D. Regular venesection is the treatment of choice.
   E. An arthritis, due to urate deposition in the affected joints, may be a feature.
   F. Splenomegaly is unusual.

161. The following are true of Wilson's disease:
   A. Serum caeruloplasmin levels are elevated.
   B. Treatment with D-penicillamine slows down progression of the liver disease.
   C. Urinary copper excretion is high.
   D. Deposits of copper in the lens of the eye give rise to the characteristic Kayser–Fleischer rings.
   E. The disease may present in chidhood as an acute, fulminant hepatitis.
   F. Heterozygous individuals are usually asymptomatic.

(Answers overleaf)

159. A. True. The reason for female predominance is unknown.
  B. False. Antimitochondrial antibodies are detectable in 95% of cases; anti-smooth muscle antibodies are found in autoimmune chronic active hepatitis.
  C. False. Abdominal pain is unusual.
  D. False. They are of no benefit and may exacerbate osteoporosis.
  E. True. The peak incidence occurs in this age group.
  F. False. An association with HLA-DR8 has been reported; HLA-A3 is increased in idiopathic haemochromatosis.

160. A. False. There is raised ferritin, reflecting increased iron stores.
  B. True. It produces the classical 'slate-grey' appearance.
  C. False. This is a primary, genetically determined disease; cf. haemosiderosis.
  D. True. This depletes the body's iron stores.
  E. False. The arthritis is due to calcium pyrophosphate deposition (pseudogout).
  F. True. However, hepatomegaly is almost invariable.

161. A. False. Caeruloplasmin levels are low.
  B. True. It is a chelating agent; liver function improves if this agent is given early on.
  C. True. It rises further on administration of D-penicillamine.
  D. False. The deposits are in the cornea.
  E. True. It may also present with neurological features.
  F. True. Heterozygotes remain in zero copper balance.

162. In liver failure due to cirrhosis:

A. The ascites is best managed by a thiazide diuretic.

B. Sclerotherapy should not be used for the acute treatment of variceal haemorrhage.

C. Anorexia is a common symptom of impending encephalopathy.

D. Encephalopathy is usually improved by a surgical porto-systemic shunt procedure.

E. Plasma volume and cardiac output are increased in most patients with ascites.

F. Lactulose improves the encephalopathy by inhibiting the growth of colonic ammonia-producing bacteria.

163. Hepatic granulomata:

A. Are a feature of sarcoidosis.

B. May be seen in Crohn's disease.

C. Usually cause jaundice.

D. Usually cause hepatomegaly.

E. Are a feature of primary biliary cirrhosis.

F. May be caused by treatment with sulphonamides.

164. In pyogenic liver abscess:

A. The patient may present with pyrexia of unknown origin.

B. There is usually a lymphocytosis.

C. The causative organisms are frequently anaerobes.

D. The diagnosis is suggested by the finding of raised transaminases on routine liver function testing.

E. Abscesses are more common in the right lobe of the liver than the left.

F. A 1-week course of intravenous antibiotics is usually curative.

(Answers overleaf)

162. A. False. Spironolactone is the diuretic of choice; thiazides exacerbate potassium depletion.
  B. False. A vasopressin infusion or a Sengstaken–Blakemore tube are alternatives.
  C. True. Reversal of sleep pattern is another common symptom.
  D. False. Such a procedure may exacerbate the encephalopathy.
  E. True. This is possibly due to raised plasma renin and aldosterone levels.
  F. True. It also clears the bacteria through its purgative action.

163. A. True. This is one of the commonest causes in the UK.
  B. True. This is a less common cause.
  C. False. The bilirubin is usually normal, but alkaline phosphatase is raised.
  D. True. There is usually a moderate enlargement.
  E. True. However, they are more commonly seen in systemic rather than primary hepatic diseases.
  F. True. Many different drugs can cause them.

164. A. True. Abdominal pain and hepatomegaly may be absent.
  B. False. There is a neutrophilia.
  C. True. *Streptococcus milleri* is the causative organism in up to 50% of cases.
  D. False. Raised alkaline phosphatase is suggestive.
  E. True. The reason is unknown.
  F. False. Six weeks of antibiotics and surgical or percutaneous drainage are required in most cases.

19. Endocrine diseases

165. The following statements are true:

A. Circulating thyroxine is mostly unbound to plasma proteins.

B. Parathyroid hormone and calcitonin are both glycoproteins.

C. Human chorionic gonadotrophin and luteinising hormone are structurally related.

D. ACTH stimulates its target cell by binding to cell-surface receptors.

E. Cell receptors for vitamin D are located in the cytoplasm and nucleus.

F. Oestradiol inhibits the expression of cell receptors for progesterone.

166. Adrenocorticotrophic hormone (ACTH):

A. Is synthesised by pituitary somatotroph cells.

B. Peak secretion occurs just before waking.

C. Possesses melanocyte stimulating activity.

D. Is the principal regulator of aldosterone secretion.

E. Synthesis and release is controlled by corticotrophin releasing hormone (CRH) acting synergistically with antidiuretic hormone (ADH).

F. Somatostatin inhibits release by the pituitary.

167. The following are recognised causes of anterior pituitary hypofunction:

A. Tuberculous meningitis.

B. Craniospinal radiation.

C. Severe head injury.

D. Hypotension during pregnancy.

E. Wegener's granulomatosis.

F. Defective diaphragma sellae.

(Answers overleaf)

165. **A.** **False.** The free fraction constitutes less than 1% of total circulating thyroxine.
    B. **False.** They are both polypeptides.
    C. **True.** Both are two-subunit glycated polypeptides, with α- and β-subunits of very similar amino acid sequence and bind them to the receptor.
    D. **True.** ACTH binds to a cell-surface receptor, using cyclic AMP as a secondary messenger.
    E. **True.** As for all steroid hormones.
    F. **False.** Oestradiol (and its synthetic counterparts) induce expression of the progesterone receptor, for example, in breast cancer cells.

166. **A.** **False.** Synthesised by pituitary corticotroph cells.
    B. **True.**
    C. **True.** This accounts for the increased pigmentation of skin and buccal mucosa seen in primary hypoadrenalism and Nelson's syndrome.
    D. **False.** Aldosterone secretion by the adrenal cortex is regulated principally by the renin–angiotensin system.
    E. **True.**
    F. **False.** Somatostatin has no known effect on ACTH release.

167. **A.** **True.** Damage to the hypothalamus or pituitary.
    B. **True.**
    C. **True.** Causing stalk damage.
    D. **True.** This is Sheehan's syndrome, most commonly associated with postpartum haemorrhage, but also caused by antepartum haemorrhage, or other causes of hypotension during pregnancy.
    E. **False.** Hypopituitarism is associated with various granulomatous diseases, e.g. tuberculosis, sarcoid and eosinophilic granuloma, but not Wegener's.
    F. **True.** Assumed to be the cause of empty sella syndrome.

168. In the investigation of suspected hypopituitarism:

A. Basal hormone measurements are rarely of value.

B. The insulin tolerance test is safe in patients with heart disease.

C. Glucocorticoid replacement should not be commenced until the results of serum cortisol measurements are known.

D. Air encephalography is usually the technique of choice for definitive radiology of the pituitary.

E. Glucagon can be used to assess growth hormone response.

F. LHRH and TRH tests can be performed simultaneously with an insulin tolerance test.

169. In the treatment of hypopituitarism:

A. Thyroid hormone replacement should be started before glucocorticoid replacement.

B. Cyclical oestrogen replacement will usually restore fertility in women of child-bearing age.

C. Oestrogen unopposed by progesterone should not be given to women with a uterus.

D. Androgen replacement is usually contraindicated in elderly men.

E. Occult cranial diabetes insipidus may be unmasked by glucocorticoid replacement therapy.

F. Women with Sheehan's syndrome usually require desmopressin (DDAVP).

(Answers overleaf)

168. A. **False.** Much can be learnt from basal measurements of hormones secreted by the pituitary and target organs, e.g. cortisol, thyroxine, LH, FSH, testosterone (men), oestradiol (women) and prolactin.

B. **False.** Contraindicated in elderly patients and those with epilepsy. Potentially hazardous in children.

C. **False.** In suspected hypoadrenalism (primary or secondary) glucocorticoid replacement should be started immediately after a blood sample for cortisol and ACTH has been taken. After stabilising the patient's condition, the glucocorticoid replacement can be temporarily withdrawn to facilitate more detailed investigation.

D. **False.** High-resolution computerised tomography and MRI scanning are the most widely used techniques.

E. **True.**

F. **True.** As a 'combined pituitary function test'.

169. A. **False.** Glucocorticoid replacement should always be started before thyroid hormone replacement.

B. **False.** Restoration of fertility requires gonadotrophin (hCG and FSH) therapy, or the administration of pulsatile GnRH (given subcutaneously by pump).

C. **True.** There is an increased risk of endometrial carcinoma.

D. **False.** Androgen replacement in men is appropriate for all ages, to maintain bone marrow function, skeletal muscle strength and libido, if desired.

E. **True.** Cortisol permits renal clearance of free water.

F. **False.** Sheehan's syndrome usually requires anterior pituitary replacement therapy only.

170. Isolated growth hormone deficiency in children:

  A. Is associated with an early puberty.
  B. Is a recognised cause of neonatal hypoglycaemia.
  C. Can be confirmed by basal measurements of growth hormone.
  D. Can be treated effectively by intranasal growth hormone replacement.
  E. Can be caused by Jakob–Creutzfeldt disease.
  F. Is a cause of Laron-type dwarfism.

171. The following are recognised features of acromegaly:

  A. Hypertension.
  B. Carpal tunnel syndrome.
  C. Hepatosplenomegaly.
  D. Osteoporosis.
  E. Multinodular goitre.
  F. Galactorrhoea.

172. The following treatments are used in acromegaly:

  A. Bromocriptine.
  B. Trans-sphenoidal surgery.
  C. External pituitary irradiation.
  D. Metyrapone.
  E. Somatostatin analogue (octreotide).
  F. Desmopressin.

(Answers overleaf)

170. **A.** **False.** Puberty is typically delayed.
   B. **True.**
   C. **False.** Provocative dynamic testing with insulin, glucagon or arginine is required to confirm the diagnosis biochemically.
   D. **False.** GH is best given by subcutaneous injection, at least three times per week.
   E. **False.** Cases of Jakob–Creutzfeldt disease have been linked to treatment with GH prepared from autopsy pituitaries, leading to a halt in treatment until biosynthetic human GH became available.
   F. **False.** This is caused by target-organ insensitivity to GH, and is characterised by high GH levels, but low levels of somatomedin C (IGF-1).

171. **A.** **True.**
   B. **True.**
   C. **True.** As part of a generalised organomegaly.
   D. **False.** Effects on the skeleton include kyphosis and secondary osteoarthritis.
   E. **True.** About one-quarter of patients have a goitre, commonly multinodular.
   F. **True.** Some GH secreting tumours also secrete prolactin and will cause galactorrhoea in women.

172. **A.** **True.**
   B. **True.** In suitable patients this is the most effective treatment; it can be curative if small tumours are selectively resected and pituitary function preserved.
   C. **True.** Carefully planned external pituitary irradiation is an effective treatment, but it takes several years to exert its effects (50% reduction in mean GH level every 2 years).
   D. **False.** This is useful in the medical treatment of Cushing's syndrome.
   E. **True.** Native somatostatin is effective in suppressing GH secretion in acromegaly, but its clinical usefulness is restricted by its very short half-life. The long-acting somatostatin analogue octreotide is an effective treatment, administered by subcutaneous injection (b.d. or t.d.s.) or depot formulation.
   F. **False.** Desmopressin (DDAVP) is used in diabetes insipidus.

173. Causes of an elevated serum hCG include:

A. Seminoma of the testis.

B. Hepatocellular carcinoma.

C. Choriocarcinoma.

D. Hydatidiform mole.

E. Bronchial carcinoma.

F. Cranial germinoma.

174. The following are recognised causes of hyperprolactinaemia:

A. Normal pregnancy.

B. Combined oral contraceptive pill.

C. Hyperthyroidism.

D. Chlorpheniramine.

E. Craniopharyngioma.

F. Herpes zoster infection of a thoracic dermatome.

175. Prolactin-secreting microadenomas of the pituitary (microprolactinomas):

A. Are present in up to 20% of the adult population.

B. Can usually be treated with bromocriptine.

C. Often cause visual field defects.

D. In women, are less common than macroprolactinomas.

E. Do not require treatment in amenorrhoeic women not desiring fertility.

F. Seldom require treatment by pituitary surgery.

(Answers overleaf)

173. A. **True.** All germ cell tumours secrete hCG and α-fetoprotein (AFP).
     B. **True.** Although AFP is the most useful tumour marker.
     C. **True.**
     D. **True.**
     E. **True.**
     F. **True.** Another germ cell tumour.

174. A. **True.** Oestrogen stimulates growth of pituitary lactotrophs.
     B. **True.** The oestrogen component can cause modest hyperprolactinaemia.
     C. **False.** Primary *hypo*thyroidism can cause hyperprolactinaemia, probably through increased TRH secretion.
     D. **False.** Many drugs can cause hyperprolactinaemia, through inhibition of dopamine action (e.g. chlorpromazine) or secretion (e.g. methyldopa, H_2-receptor blockers).
     E. **True.** Hypothalamic tumours interfere with dopamine secretion, thereby causing disinhibition of prolactin secretion by lactotrophs.
     F. **True.** As may other persistent sensory stimuli to the chest wall or nipple.

175. A. **False.** They are found in 5–10% of adults but most are not diagnosed.
     B. **True.** Bromocriptine is highly effective in most cases at suppressing the serum prolactin, leading to the resumption of normal menses.
     C. **False.** Microadenomas are, by definition, less than one centimetre in diameter, and they 'never' cause visual field defects or other pressure effects, e.g. hypopituitarism.
     D. **False.** About 80% of prolactinomas in women are microadenomas.
     E. **False.** Such women are oestrogen-deficient and therefore at risk of osteoporosis in later life.
     F. **True.**

176. The syndrome of inappropriate secretion of ADH:

A. Causes a high serum sodium concentration.

B. Causes an inappropriately high urine osmolality.

C. May be caused by overtreatment with diuretics.

D. Can be treated with fluid restriction alone.

E. May respond to treatment with demeclocycline.

F. Is usually caused by ectopic secretion of ADH.

177. The following statements are true of thyroid hormones:

A. They are synthesised and secreted by the parafollicular cells.

B. The principal thyroid hormone secreted by the thyroid gland is thyroxine.

C. Tri-iodothyronine (T3) is the most biologically active thyroid hormone.

D. The protein-bound fraction of circulating thyroxine is not biologically active.

E. T3 binds to thyroxine binding globulin (TBG) with higher affinity than thyroxine.

F. Total circulating T3 levels rise during pregnancy.

178. The following are recognised features of hypothyroidism in adults:

A. Carpal tunnel syndrome.

B. Pretibial myxoedema.

C. Pericardial effusion.

D. Hypercholesterolaemia.

E. Hyponatraemia.

F. Cerebellar ataxia.

179. The following are true of autoimmune thyroid disease:

A. Hyperthyroidism can occur in Hashimoto's thyroiditis.

B. Men are more commonly affected than women.

C. There is an association with pernicious anaemia.

D. The highest titres of anti-thyroid peroxidase antibodies are found in atrophic thyroiditis.

E. The condition is excluded by the absence of anti-thyroid peroxidase.

F. Circulating antibodies may block the TSH receptor.

(Answers overleaf)

176. A. False. ⎱ The hallmark of excessive ADH secretion is a low
serum sodium concentration associated with an
   B. True. ⎰ inappropriately high urine osmolality (greater
than 150 mosmol/kg) in a patient who is
   C. False. ⎰ not volume depleted.
   D. True.   And correction of the underlying cause.
   E. True.
   F. False.   Only small cell carcinoma of the bronchus is ever
associated with true ectopic tumour production of ADH.

177. A. False.   They are synthesised and secreted by the follicular
cells. The parafollicular (or C cells) secrete calcitonin.
   B. True. ⎱ Thyroxine is converted enzymatically to T3
   C. True. ⎰ (or reverse T3) in the liver and other tissues.
   D. True.   Only the free (unbound) fraction is biologically
active on target cells.
   E. False.   T3 has a lower affinity for TBG. This substantially
affects the ratio of free T4/free T3 (about 5:1) compared to
total circulating T4/T3 (about 50:1).
   F. True.   Also total T4 levels, due to an oestrogen-induced rise
in TBG.

178. A. True.
   B. False.   A feature of Graves' disease.
   C. True.   Effusions may occur into any serous cavity.
   D. True.   This predisposes to vascular atheroma.
   E. True.   Due to inappropriate secretion of ADH.
   F. True.   A rare complication.

179. A. True.   There may be a phase of mild hyperthyroidism, due
to TSH receptor stimulating antibodies.
   B. False.   Women are affected about five times more than men.
   C. True.   There is an association with other organ-specific
autoimmune disorders such as Addison's disease, vitiligo and
IDDM.
   D. False.   Very high titres indicate Hashimoto's thyroiditis.
   E. False.   Up to 15% of patients with autoimmune thyroid
disease do not have anti-TPO antibodies.
   F. True.   Causing hypothyroidism, although the principal
mechanism for this is the destructive effect of cell-mediated
autoimmunity and cytotoxic autoantibodies.

180. The following are recognised features of thyrotoxicosis:

   A. Atrial fibrillation.
   B. Proximal myopathy.
   C. Hypocalcaemia.
   D. Gynaecomastia.
   E. Neuropathy.
   F. Osteoporosis.

181. Primary malignant tumours of the thyroid:

   A. Often present as localised swellings (solitary nodules).
   B. Usually show normal uptake on isotope scanning.
   C. Are excluded if a cystic lesion is shown on ultrasound scanning.
   D. Which have metastasised may be treatable by ^{131}I.
   E. May be associated with a family history of Zollinger–Ellison syndrome.
   F. Anaplastic carcinomas are commonest in young adults.

182. The following may be features of primary hypoadrenalism:

   A. Hypertension.
   B. Hypoglycaemia.
   C. Hypokalaemia.
   D. Abdominal pain.
   E. Fever.
   F. Calcification on plain abdominal X-ray.

183. Recognised features of Cushing's syndrome include:

   A. Hirsutism.
   B. Depression.
   C. Osteomalacia.
   D. Proximal myopathy.
   E. Hypokalaemia.
   F. Hypercalcaemia.

(Answers overleaf)

180. A. **True.**
 B. **True.**
 C. **False.**   But *hyper*calcaemia is a recognised feature.
 D. **True.**
 E. **False.**
 F. **True.**

181. A. **True.**
 B. **False.**   Typically, they appear as 'cold' areas on isotope scans.
 C. **False.**   Some carcinomas are cystic.
 D. **True.**   Metastatic, follicular and papillary carcinoma.
 E. **False.**   Medullary cell carcinoma is associated with phaeochromocytoma in multiple endocrine neoplasia (MEN) type 2, but Zollinger–Ellison syndrome (usually due to pancreatic gastrinoma) is a feature of MEN type 1.
 F. **False.**   Commonest in the elderly.

182. A. **False.**   *Hypo*tension is a feature of severe hypoadrenalism.
 B. **True.**
 C. **False.**   *Hyper*kalaemia is a feature, due to mineralocorticoid deficiency.
 D. **True.**   One of several non-specific gastrointestinal symptoms found in Addisonian crises.
 E. **True.**   A feature of Addisonian crisis.
 F. **True.**   Adrenal calcification suggests tuberculosis.

183. A. **True.**   Due at least partly to increased adrenal androgens. The role of glucocorticoids is uncertain.
 B. **True.**   Also psychosis.
 C. **False.**   Osteo*porosis* results from prolonged glucocorticoid excess.
 D. **True.**
 E. **True.**   Although the serum potassium is often in the normal range in Cushing's syndrome, hypokalaemia may be a prominent feature of ectopic ACTH syndrome due to malignant tumours, e.g. small cell bronchial carcinoma.
 F. **False.**

184. Phaeochromocytomas:

- **A.** Are the underlying cause of 5% of cases of hypertension.
- **B.** Usually arise from the adrenal cortex.
- **C.** Are usually malignant.
- **D.** Are most commonly diagnosed at post-mortem.
- **E.** Predominantly secrete noradrenaline.
- **F.** May be associated with primary hyperparathyroidism.

185. The following are recognised causes of hypogonadism in adult men:

- **A.** Klinefelter's syndrome.
- **B.** Measles.
- **C.** Dystrophia myotonica.
- **D.** Kallmann's syndrome.
- **E.** Haemochromatosis.
- **F.** Anorexia nervosa.

186. The following are causes of secondary amenorrhoea:

- **A.** Gonadal dysgenesis.
- **B.** Marathon running.
- **C.** Anorexia nervosa.
- **D.** Cytotoxic chemotherapy.
- **E.** Polycystic ovary syndrome.
- **F.** Hypothyroidism.

187. Clinical features of 45,XO Turner's syndrome include:

- **A.** Primary amenorrhoea.
- **B.** Ambiguous genitalia.
- **C.** Patent ductus arteriosus.
- **D.** Osteoporosis.
- **E.** Final height usually below 5 ft.
- **F.** Horseshoe kidney.

188. The following are recognised causes of gynaecomastia:

- **A.** Klinefelter's syndrome.
- **B.** Normal puberty.
- **C.** Amiloride.
- **D.** Cannabis.
- **E.** Seminoma of the testis.
- **F.** Thyrotoxicosis.

(Answers overleaf)

184. A. **False.** About 1 in 1000 of cases of hypertension is the figure usually quoted.
     B. **False.** The adrenal *medulla* is the location of 90%, and 10% are extra-adrenal.
     C. **False.** About 10% are malignant.
     D. **True.** Up to three-quarters of all phaeochromocytomas.
     E. **True.**
     F. **True.** In MEN 2.

185. A. **True.** Primary hypogonadism.
     B. **False.** Mumps orchitis can cause primary hypogonadism.
     C. **True.** Primary hypogonadism.
     D. **True.** Isolated GnRH deficiency and anosmia.
     E. **True.**
     F. **True.** Hypogonadotrophic hypogonadism.

186. A. **False.** Causes *primary* amenorrhoea only.
     B. **True.** ⎫
     C. **True.** ⎬ Through relative GnRH deficiency.
     D. **True.**
     E. **True.**
     F. **True.** Caused by hyperprolactinaemia.

187. A. **True.**
     B. **False.** Genitalia are normal female.
     C. **False.** Cardiac abnormalities include coarctation of the aorta, bicuspid aortic valve and aortic stenosis.
     D. **True.** Caused by oestrogen deficiency.
     E. **True.**
     F. **True.** Renal tract abnormalities are common.

188. A. **True.** Due to hypogonadism.
     B. **True.** Very common, can be regarded as physiological.
     C. **False.**
     D. **True.** Direct oestrogenic effect.
     E. **True.** Caused by increased oestrogen production, stimulated by tumour secretion of hCG.
     F. **True.**

20. Metabolic bone disease and mineral metabolism

189. The following are true of osteoporosis:

- **A.** A specific underlying cause can be identified in most cases.
- **B.** Routine plasma biochemistry is usually normal.
- **C.** Osteoporosis is characterised by an increased quantity of unmineralised bone matrix.
- **D.** X-rays of long bones may show Looser's zones.
- **E.** In postmenopausal women, treatment with oestrogen is of no proven value.
- **F.** Can be caused by Conn's syndrome.

190. The following are true of osteomalacia:

- **A.** It is most commonly caused by primary phosphate deficiency.
- **B.** It rarely leads to secondary hyperparathyroidism.
- **C.** In vitamin D deficiency, plasma biochemistry typically demonstrates a low normal calcium and low phosphate.
- **D.** Patients with epilepsy have an increased incidence.
- **E.** Brown tumours of the mandible are a recognised feature.
- **F.** It is a feature of Fanconi's syndrome.

191. The following are features of idiopathic hypoparathyroidism:

- **A.** Hypophosphataemia.
- **B.** Association with Addison's disease.
- **C.** Candidiasis.
- **D.** Short stature.
- **E.** Short fourth and fifth metacarpal bones.
- **F.** Calcification of the basal ganglia.

192. The following are true of Paget's disease:

- **A.** Raised serum alkaline phosphatase reflects increased osteoclastic activity.
- **B.** Most affected individuals are asymptomatic.
- **C.** Osteogenic sarcoma arises in 15% of patients.
- **D.** Normal pressure hydrocephalus is a recognised complication.
- **E.** There is increased urinary hydroxyproline excretion.
- **F.** Calcitonin is the most effective treatment.

(Answers overleaf)

189. A. **False.**
    B. **True.** The most common exceptions to this are the cases secondary to specific endocrine disorders.
    C. **False.** This is true of osteo*malacia*.
    D. **False.** This is a feature of osteo*malacia*.
    E. **False.** Oestrogen undoubtedly reduces the rate of loss of bone mass after the menopause, and may increase bone mass in some patients.
    F. **False.** Cushing's syndrome commonly causes osteoporosis.

190. A. **False.** It is most commonly caused by vitamin D deficiency which invariably leads to secondary hyperparathyroidism; this usually keeps the plasma calcium in the low normal range and exacerbates the phosphate deficiency.
    B. **False.** (As for A, above.)
    C. **True.** (As for A, above.)
    D. **True.** Phenytoin, phenobarbitone and carbamazepine all enhance the metabolism of vitamin D, through liver enzyme induction.
    E. **False.** This is a feature of primary hyperparathyroidism.
    F. **True.** Through increased phosphaturia caused by reduced tubular phosphate reabsorption.

191. A. **False.** *Hyper*phosphataemia results from renal phosphate retention due to lack of PTH action.
    B. **True.** It is associated with organ-specific autoimmune diseases and is thought to be of autoimmune aetiology.
    C. **True.**
    D. **False.** A feature of pseudohypoparathyroidism.
    E. **False.** A feature of pseudohypoparathyroidism.
    F. **True.**

192. A. **False.** This reflects the increase in *osteoblastic* activity. Osteroclastic resorptive activity is also increased but only osteoblasts release alkaline phosphate.
    B. **True.**
    C. **False.** Probably arises in less than 1% of cases.
    D. **False.** *Obstructive* hydrocephalus is a recognised complication.
    E. **True.** Reflects increased bone resorption due to increased osteoclastic activity.
    F. **False.** Calcitonin was the most effective treatment for some years, but it has been superseded by the bisphosphonates pamidronate (APD) and clodronate.

21. Diabetes mellitus and diseases of lipid and intermediary metabolism

193. The following are true of fat and carbohydrate metabolism:

A. Glucagon is secreted by the δ cells of the islets of Langerhans.

B. C peptide is the precursor molecule for insulin.

C. Peripheral lipolysis is promoted by glucagon.

D. Insulin promotes storage of glucagon by the liver.

E. In prolonged starvation, ketone bodies become the main source of energy.

F. Gluconeogenesis is inhibited by glucagon.

194. In insulin-dependent diabetes mellitus (IDDM):

A. The genetic susceptibility to the condition is linked to HLA-DR3 and DR4.

B. An identical twin of a child with IDDM has more than a 90% chance of developing the disease.

C. There is an extensive lymphocytic infiltration specific to the exocrine pancreas.

D. There is an increased risk of megaloblastic anaemia.

E. Circulating antibodies to insulin may be present prior to treatment with insulin.

F. There is an increased prevalence in children with congenital rubella.

195. The following are true of non-insulin-dependent diabetes (NIDDM):

A. In the UK, the highest prevalence is amongst the Asian immigrant population.

B. In women, there may be a past history of gestational diabetes.

C. It may be inherited in an autosomal dominant manner.

D. Concordance for the disease amongst identical twins is rare.

E. Macrovascular complications of diabetes are often present at the time of diagnosis.

F. Patients rarely develop microvascular complications of diabetes.

(Answers overleaf)

193. **A. False.**   It is secreted by the α cells.
   B. False.   Proinsulin is the precursor molecule which undergoes cleavage, yielding insulin and the inactive connecting peptide C peptide.
   C. True.
   D. True.
   E. True.
   F. False.   It is promoted by glucagon.

194. **A. True.**   Some 95% of people with IDDM have HLA-DR3 and/or DR4 compared to 60% of the background population.
   B. False.   Concordance in identical twins is less than 40%, suggesting that an environmental factor is necessary to trigger the disease.
   C. False.   This is specific to the *endocrine* pancreas.
   D. True.   There is an increased risk of pernicious anaemia, and other organ-specific autoimmune disorders.
   E. True.   Insulin autoantibodies may be found at presentation with IDDM, although the commonest findings are autoantibodies against the islet cells.
   F. True.   The prevalence is up to 20%.

195. **A. True.**   It is about five times more common in Asian immigrants in the UK, compared to the indigenous population.
   B. True.
   C. True.   This is particularly true in the variant of NIDDM known as maturity onset diabetes of the young (MODY).
   D. False.   Concordance for the disease amongst identical twins is more than 95%.
   E. True.   For example, ischaemic heart disease.
   F. False.

196. In drug treatment of NIDDM:

A. Chlorpropamide is a suitable choice of sulphonylurea in the elderly.

B. Metformin is the drug of choice in obese patients with NIDDM.

C. Glibenclamide can cause an alcohol-induced facial flush.

D. Metformin can cause a megaloblastic anaemia.

E. Most sulphonylureas are metabolised by the liver. T

F. Tolbutamide is suitable for patients with mild renal impairment.

197. In insulin treatment of diabetes mellitus:

A. Insulins formulated with protamine as a retarding agent are the longest acting.

B. The standard concentration of insulin in the UK is 80 units/ml.

C. Nightmares may signify nocturnal hypoglycaemia.

D. Most people with IDDM need less than 1 U/kg/day of insulin.

E. Hypoglycaemia may occur the day after strenuous exercise.

F. When mixing soluble and lente insulins in the same syringe, the soluble insulin should be drawn up first.

198. In severe diabetic ketoacidosis:

A. There is an increase in circulating free fatty acids.

B. Hypokalaemia is typically present.

C. Insulin may be given subcutaneously.

D. Intravenous bicarbonate is usually given if the arterial pH is below 6.9.

E. A neutrophil leucocytosis signifies the presence of infection.

F. Hypothermia at presentation is a poor prognostic sign.

199. The following are true of diabetic retinopathy in IDDM:

A. Almost all patients with IDDM eventually develop retinopathy.

B. Background retinopathy does not cause visual impairment.

C. Untreated proliferative retinopathy leads to blindness in 50% of eyes affected within 5 years.

D. Microaneurysms signify proliferative retinopathy.

E. Retinopathy may progress rapidly during pregnancy.

F. 'Cotton wool' spots are specific to diabetic retinopathy.

(Answers overleaf)

196. A. False. It has the longest half-life of the sulphonylurea group. Tolbutamide is the most suitable drug in this group for the elderly.
   B. True.
   C. False. This is associated with Chlorpropamide.
   D. True. Metformin inhibits vitamin B_{12} absorption, occasionally leading to megaloblastic anaemia.
   E. False. Most are cleared by the kidneys, so are contraindicated in advanced renal failure (serum creatinine rising above 250 μmol/l.).
   F. True. It is metabolised by the liver.

197. A. False. Insulins formulated with zinc are the longest acting.
   B. False. The standard concentration in the UK since 1983 has been 100 units/ml.
   C. True. Also night sweats, restlessness and morning headache.
   D. True.
   E. True.
   F. True. To avoid contaminating the vial of soluble insulin with the retarding agent, zinc.

198. A. True. Due to insulin deficiency. The free fatty acids act as substrate for the greatly increased hepatic production of ketone bodies.
   B. False. Total body potassium is invariably depleted but the serum potassium may be high, normal or low at presentation.
   C. False. This route of administration is too slow and erratic.
   D. True.
   E. False. This is a non-specific finding and is often present.
   F. True. It may respond to rewarming with a space blanket.

199. A. True. Almost all develop background retinopathy by 20 years.
   B. True. Vision is not affected until there is progression to either maculopathy or pre-proliferative retinopathy.
   C. True. Hence the importance of regular ophthalmoscopy.
   D. False. Microaneurysms are the earliest abnormality seen on ophthalmoscopy in background retinopathy.
   E. True.
   F. False. They may also be found in accelerating hypertension.

200. The following may be clinical features of diabetic neuropathy:

A. Wasting of the quadriceps muscles.
B. Loss of sinus arrhythmia.
C. Sixth nerve palsy.
D. Vomiting.
E. Atonic bladder.
F. Nocturnal diarrhoea.

201. Features of a neuropathic diabetic foot include:

A. Painful ulceration.
B. Dry skin.
C. Charcot arthropathy.
D. Cold feet.
E. Positive Romberg's sign.
F. Clawing of the toes.

202. In pregnancy complicated by IDDM:

A. Maternal mortality is comparable to that in the general population.
B. Congenital malformations are three times commoner than in non-diabetic pregnancies.
C. Babies of diabetic mothers are liable to neonatal hyperglycaemia.
D. Diabetic retinopathy usually stabilises during pregnancy.
E. There is an increased risk of pre-eclampsia.
F. Insulin requirements fall dramatically after the placenta is delivered.

(Answers overleaf)

200. A. True. A feature of diabetic amyotrophy.
 B. True. A feature of autonomic neuropathy affecting the vagus.
 C. True. Cranial and peripheral nerves may be affected by diabetic neuropathy.
 D. True. Autonomic neuropathy causing loss of gastric motility due to vagal damage.
 E. True. Loss of bladder tone due to autonomic neuropathy.
 F. True. Autonomic neuropathy.

201. A. False. Neuropathic ulcers are typically painless.
 B. True. Due to sympathetic denervation.
 C. True. Due to denervation of the joints.
 D. False. The feet can be warm, due to arteriovenous shunting.
 E. True. Due to impaired joint position sense.
 F. True. Denervation of the intrinsic muscles and unopposed action of the long extensor tendons.

202. A. True.
 B. True.
 C. False. They are liable to hypoglycaemia in the neonatal period.
 D. False. Both retinopathy and nephropathy may deteriorate rapidly, possibly secondary to improved glycaemic control.
 E. True. Also polyhydramnios, intrauterine death and macrosomia.
 F. True. Insulin requirements fall to pre-pregnancy levels.

203. In disorders of lipoprotein metabolism:

A. Severe hypercholesterolaemia can cause acute pancreatitis.

B. Dietary treatment should include an increase in the ratio of saturated to polyunsaturated fats.

C. Patients with heterozygote hereditary hypercholesterolaemia (type IIa) often die from coronary artery disease as young adults.

D. Regular exercise can increase HDL-cholesterol levels.

E. Cholestyramine is the most potent cholesterol-lowering drug.

F. Hypertriglyceridaemia may be secondary to alcohol.

204. The following are features of acute intermittent porphyria:

A. Abdominal pain.

B. Hypotension.

C. Proximal myopathy.

D. Increased urinary uroporphyrin excretion.

E. Precipitation by benzodiazepines.

F. Passage of red-brown urine.

(Answers overleaf)

203. A. False. Acute pancreatitis is a feature of severe hypertriglyceridaemia.
  B. False. Diet treatment includes the avoidance of saturated (animal) fats.
  C. False. This is true of *homo*zygote hereditary hypercholesterolaemia.
  D. True.
  E. False. The HMG–CoA reductase inhibitors, e.g. simvastatin, are the most potent drugs currently available.
  F. True.

204. A. True. With vomiting, the commonest presenting feature.
  B. False. *Hyper*tension is found in 75%.
  C. False. Sensorimotor peripheral neuropathy is found in 50%.
  D. False. This is found in porphyria cutanea tarda.
  E. False. Benzodiazepines may be used to treat epileptic seizures in acute intermittent porphyria.
  F. False. The urine turns red-brown on standing.

22. Renal and urinary disease

205. The following statements concerning the anatomy and the physiology of the kidney are true:

A. The right kidney is about 1.5 cm higher than the left.

B. The renal capsule is innervated via the T8 and T9 nerve roots.

C. Renal blood flow represents about 25% of the resting cardiac output.

D. Normal glomerular filtration rate (GFR) is about 180 litres/day.

E. Angiotensinogen is secreted by the juxtaglomerular apparatus (JGA).

F. The glomerular basement membrane forms part of the glomerular 'sieve'.

206. With regard to renal tubular function:

A. About 50% of filtered sodium is reabsorbed by the renal tubules.

B. Aldosterone increases potassium secretion by the proximal tubules.

C. The permeability of the distal tubules to water is reduced by ADH.

D. Filtered bicarbonate is mostly reabsorbed in the distal tubule.

E. Tubular calcium reabsorption is reduced by PTH.

F. The tubular reabsorptive capacity for glucose is exceeded at a plasma glucose concentration of 10 mmol/l.

205. A. False. It is 1.5 cm *lower* than the left kidney.
   B. False. It is innervated via the T10–T12, and L1 nerve roots.
   C. True.
   D. True. This is 120 ml/min.
   E. False. The JGA secretes renin.
   F. True. The other components are the capillary endothelial cells and the visceral epithelial cells of Bowman's capsule.

206. A. False. At least 99% of filtered sodium is reabsorbed.
   B. False. Aldosterone increases potassium secretion by the *distal* tubules.
   C. False. The permeability is *increased* by ADH, so that water moves from the tubular lumen to the hyperosmolar medullary interstitium.
   D. False. Some 80–90% of filtered bicarbonate is reabsorbed in the *proximal* tubule.
   E. False. Tubular reabsorption of calcium is *increased* by PTH.
   F. True.

207. The following are true of proteinuria:

A. The urinary protein excretion rate is usually decreased in the upright posture.

B. A urinary protein excretion rate of > 250 mg per day is usually of pathological significance.

C. Bence-Jones proteinuria can be detected by the salicylsulphonic acid test.

D. Heavy proteinuria (more than 3 g/24 h) is usually of tubular origin.

E. Mild proteinuria may be found in essential hypertension.

F. Heavy proteinuria may be a feature of pre-eclampsia.

208. Causes of polyuria include the following:

A. Diabetes mellitus.

B. Chronic renal failure.

C. Hypoadrenalism.

D. Hypercalcaemia.

E. Hypokalaemia.

F. Lithium carbonate therapy.

209. The following are recognised causes of acute nephritic syndrome:

A. Bacterial endocarditis.

B. Idiopathic thrombocytopenic purpura.

C. Epstein–Barr virus.

D. Gonococcus.

E. Goodpasture's syndrome.

F. *Plasmodium vivax.*

210. Causes of chronic renal failure include:

A. Amyloidosis.

B. Rheumatoid arthritis.

C. Hypertension.

D. Unilateral renal artery stenosis.

E. Sarcoidosis.

F. Henoch–Schönlein purpura.

(Answers overleaf)

207. **A.** **False.** This is usually *increased* in the upright posture, and may lead to abnormally high protein measurements on random samples in normal ambulant patients (orthostatic proteinuria).
   B. **True.**
   C. **True.**
   D. **False.** It is always of glomerular origin.
   E. **True.** But only when severe or in the accelerated phase.
   F. **True.**

208. **A.** **True.** Osmotic diuresis due to high concentration of filtered glucose.
   B. **True.** Osmotic diuresis due to high concentration of filtered urea.
   C. **False.**
   D. **True.**⎫
   E. **True.** ⎬ Nephrogenic diabetes insipidus.
   F. **True.** ⎭

209. **A.** **True.**
   B. **False.**
   C. **True.**
   D. **False.**
   E. **True.**
   F. **False.** *Plasmodium falciparum.*

210. **A.** **True.**
   B. **True.** Although drugs used in the treatment of rheumatoid arthritis, e.g. gold and penicillamine, are the commoner causes of nephropathy.
   C. **True.** Hypertensive nephrosclerosis.
   D. **False.** Bilateral renal artery sclerosis can lead to CRF.
   E. **True.** Interstitial nephropathy.
   F. **True.**

211. The anaemia of chronic renal failure:

A. Is partly due to shortened red cell survival.

B. Responds to treatment with synthetic human erythropoietin.

C. Improves rapidly after successful renal transplantation.

D. Usually responds to vitamin B_{12} supplementation.

E. Improves after nephrectomy in patients with end-stage renal disease.

F. Is less severe in patients with polycystic kidney disease.

212. The following may be features of advanced uraemia:

A. Pancreatitis.

B. Kussmaul breathing.

C. Metabolic alkalosis.

D. Hypertriglyceridaemia.

E. Cardiomyopathy.

F. Myoclonus.

213. Causes of nephrotic syndrome include:

A. Indomethacin.

B. Hepatitis A.

C. Multiple myeloma.

D. Intravenous drug abuse.

E. Hodgkin's disease.

F. Gold treatment.

214. In acute post-streptococcal glomerulonephritis:

A. The preceding infection is usually in the lower gastrointestinal tract.

B. There is usually a latency of 3 months or more.

C. Group A, type 12 β-haemolytic streptococci are the usual causative organisms.

D. Nephrotic syndrome is the usual clinical presentation.

E. A low serum C3 is often found.

F. Acute renal failure is rarely severe enough to require temporary dialysis.

(Answers overleaf)

211. A. **True.**
     B. **True.**
     C. **True.** Rapid restoration of normal erythropoietin production.
     D. **False.** Iron deficiency is common, due to malabsorption, marginal dietary intake and increased mucosal blood loss. Dietary folate intake may also be marginal.
     E. **False.** Anaemia is usually more severe in nephrectomised patients, presumably due to complete deficiency of erythropoietin.
     F. **True.** Erythropoietin production is better maintained in polycystic kidney disease.

212. A. **True.**
     B. **True.** Respiratory compensation for metabolic acidosis.
     C. **False.**
     D. **True.** Very-low-density lipoproteins are also increased in uraemia, high-density lipoproteins are decreased.
     E. **True.**
     F. **True.** One of many effects of uraemia on the central nervous system.

213. A. **True.** It also causes tubulointestinal aephnopathy.
     B. **False.** Hepatitis B is a cause.
     C. **True.**
     D. **True.**
     E. **True.**
     F. **True.**

214. A. **False.** Usually the upper respiratory tract.
     B. **False.** Usually 1–3 weeks.
     C. **True.**
     D. **False.** Typically presents as acute nephritic syndrome.
     E. **True.** With variable reduction of C_2, C_4 and C1q, probably due to alternative pathway activation.
     F. **True.**

215. IgA nephropathy (Berger's disease):

A. Typically presents as recurrent macroscopic haematuria.

B. Is commonest in young adult men.

C. Is a cause of sterile pyuria.

D. Usually responds to steroids.

E. Does not progress to chronic renal failure.

F. Mesangial deposits of IgA in the glomeruli are characteristic.

216. Minimal change nephropathy:

A. Is usually accompanied by hypertension.

B. Usually progresses to chronic renal failure.

C. Renal biopsy is mandatory.

D. Usually responds to steroids.

E. Fusion of the epithelial cell foot processes on electron microscopy is characteristic.

F. Initial failure to respond to steroids is of no prognostic significance.

217. In diabetic nephropathy:

A. The incidence is unrelated to the duration of diabetes.

B. Progression to chronic renal failure is rare.

C. Intensive treatment of coexistent hypertension may retard progression of renal failure.

D. 'Dipstick' positive proteinuria signifies irreversibility of the condition.

E. Nodular glomerulosclerosis (Kimmelstiel–Wilson lesion) is the usual finding on renal biopsy.

F. The GFR may be supranormal.

218. The following drug or toxin can cause the stated renal disease:

A. Penicillamine and nephrotic syndrome.

B. Penicillin and acute interstitial nephropathy.

C. Paracetamol and acute renal failure.

D. Mercury and nephrogenic diabetes insipidus.

E. X-ray contrast media and acute tubular necrosis (ATN).

F. Organic gold and acute tubular necrosis.

(Answers overleaf)

215. A. **True.** Sometimes accompanied by loin pain.
    B. **True.**
    C. **False.** Red cells, cellular casts and proteinuria are the usual findings in the urine.
    D. **False.** In many cases the lesion is benign, and observation only is required. No treatment has been shown to alter the course of the progressive or relapsing disease.
    E. **False.**
    F. **True.** Renal biopsy is nearly always performed to establish the diagnosis with certainty.

216. A. **False.** Hypertension is rare.
    B. **False.** This is very rare.
    C. **False.** But it may be needed to confirm or refute diagnosis if resistant to stenosis.
    D. **True.** There is an 80–90% response rate.
    E. **True.** However, this appearance is not specific for minimal change and is seen in many other glomerular diseases. Nevertheless, in conjunction with normal glomeruli on light microscopy, these findings are diagnostic of minimal change nephropathy.
    F. **False.** This suggests a less favourable long-term outcome.

217. A. **False.**
    B. **False.** Deterioration of renal function is inevitable, although the rate is unpredictable.
    C. **True.**
    D. **True.**
    E. **False.** Diffuse glomerulosclerosis is the commonest finding, although it is not specific to diabetes mellitus.
    F. **True.** Hyperfiltration with raised GFR appears to be the earliest stage of diabetic nephropathy, and there is some evidence that the condition may be reversible at this stage, if tight glycaemic control can be achieved.

218. A. **True.**
    B. **True.** A hypersensitivity reaction.
    C. **True.** Although hepatic toxicity usually predominates.
    D. **False.** Causes acute renal failure.
    E. **True.** But usually only when there is pre-existing renal disease, especially diabetes. Reduced circulatory volume is a predisposing factor.
    F. **False.** Causes nephrotic syndrome.

219. Adult polycystic kidney disease:

   A. Is inherited as an autosomal recessive condition.

   B. Can lead to end-stage renal failure.

   C. Requires renal biopsy for confirmation of diagnosis.

   D. Is often associated with hepatic cysts.

   E. Is associated with an increased incidence of subarachnoid haemorrhage.

   F. May be complicated by renal tract calculi.

220. The following are true of urinary tract infection:

   A. Commonest in men.

   B. Skin commensals are the usual causative organisms.

   C. In pregnancy, is more likely to lead to pyelonephritis.

   D. May be the first sign of a bladder tumour.

   E. A 5-day course of antibiotic therapy is usually adequate.

   F. May lead to papillary necrosis in patients with diabetes.

221. Tuberculosis of the urinary tract:

   A. Is a cause of sterile pyuria.

   B. Can be confidently excluded if no AFBs are seen on microscopic examination of at least three early morning specimens of urine.

   C. A pulmonary focus is almost always present.

   D. May lead to tuberculous epididymitis.

   E. Rarely causes any direct renal damage.

   F. May be complicated by urinary tract obstruction.

222. The following are true of urinary tract stones:

   A. Uric acid stones are radio-opaque.

   B. Pyonephrosis is a recognised complication.

   C. Occurring in patients with hypercalciuria, it is usually secondary to hypercalcaemia.

   D. Renal and ureteric colic are nearly always accompanied by haematuria.

   E. Patients with idiopathic hypercalciuria may benefit from treatment with thiazide diuretics.

   F. Patients with uric acid stones should be treated with allopurinol.

(Answers overleaf)

219. A. False. Autosomal dominant with 100% penetrance.
  B. True. Accounts for 5–10% of all cases of end-stage renal disease.
  C. False. This is inappropriate. In advanced cases the diagnosis is readily made clinically, confirmed on ultrasound. Difficulty arises with the detection of early cases, e.g. screening of young members of affected families.
  D. True. About 30% of cases.
  E. True. Some 10–22% of patients may have intracranial aneurysms.
  F. True.

220. A. False. Commonest in women.
  B. False. Faecal organisms predominate.
  C. True.
  D. True.
  E. True.
  F. True. Papillary necrosis is a complication of severe acute pyelonephritis and is more common in patients with diabetes.

221. A. True.
  B. False. If no AFBs are seen on microscopy, active infection can be excluded only by culture of at least three early morning urine specimens, for 6 weeks.
  C. True. Tuberculosis of the urinary tract results from haematogenous spread.
  D. True. Also the bladder (tuberculous cystitis).
  E. False. A progressive interstitial nephropathy develops with extensive fibrosis and distortion of the gross anatomy of the kidney, which can lead to irreversible chronic renal failure.
  F. True. Through stricture formation.

221. A. False.
  B. True. Acute infection above an obstructing stone.
  C. False. Most patients with hypercalciuria have idiopathic hypercalciuria and are not hypercalcaemic.
  D. True. May be macroscopic or microscopic.
  E. True. Thiazides reduce urinary calcium excretion.
  F. True.

223. The following are true of urinary tract obstruction:

    A. Renal failure implies that both kidneys are obstructed.

    B. The passage of normal volumes of urine excludes obstruction.

    C. Can be caused by carcinoma of the cervix.

    D. Relief of the obstruction may be followed by a diuresis.

    E. The earliest indication of reduced renal function is a fall in glomerular filtration rate.

    F. Acute obstruction is more likely to cause irreversible renal damage than is slowly progressive obstruction.

224. Adenocarcinoma of the kidney:

    A. Has an increased incidence in cigarette smokers.

    B. Is usually operable at presentation.

    C. Rarely causes hypercalcaemia.

    D. Is a cause of polycythaemia.

    E. Is highly responsive to chemotherapy.

    F. Is associated with retinal haemangioblastoma.

(Answers overleaf)

223. A. True. It may also imply obstruction of a solitary functioning kidney.

B. False. Complete obstruction of the urinary tract will cause anuria, but the patient with partial obstruction will continue to pass normal, or even increased, volumes of urine.

C. True. Can be caused by any form of pelvic malignancy.

D. True. This is usually short-lived and reflects previous salt and water overload and an osmotic diuresis resulting from high plasma urea concentration. There may sometimes be a temporary concentrating defect leading to inappropriate salt and water loss.

E. False. Urinary concentrating ability and acidification are the earliest functions to be compromised.

F. False. Acute obstruction is usually associated with pain, leading to an earlier presentation than is the case with a slowly progressive obstruction, which is likely to be pain-free.

224. A. True. It is also three times commoner in men.

B. True. In 60–70% of cases.

C. False. Humoral hypercalcaemia of malignancy is common.

D. True. Due to excess erythropoietin production by tumour.

E. False. Chemotherapy is of little value.

F. True. Von Hippel–Lindau syndrome.

23. Salt and water homeostasis and acid–base balance

225. The following are recognised causes of diabetes insipidus:

A. Hypoadrenalism.
B. Hypercalcaemia.
C. Lithium carbonate.
D. Histiocytosis X.
E. Carbamazepine.
F. DIDMOAD syndrome.

226. Causes of hyponatraemia include the following:

A. Hyperglycaemia.
B. Hyperlipidaemia.
C. Renal failure.
D. Chlorpropamide.
E. Chlorpromazine.
F. Demethylchlortetracycline.

227. Causes of hypokalaemia include the following:

A. Spironolactone.
B. Captopril.
C. Conn's syndrome.
D. Carbenoxolone.
E. Adrenal replacement therapy.
F. Renal tubular acidosis type 4.

228. The following are true of acid–base homeostasis:

A. Intracellular pH is held within the narrow limits of pH 7.38–7.42.
B. Important buffer systems include red cell haemoglobin.
C. In acute respiratory acidosis, renal conservation of bicarbonate occurs within 8–12 hours.
D. Doxapram can cause an acute respiratory acidosis.
E. The anion gap is normal in diabetic ketoacidosis.
F. The anion gap is increased in lactic acidosis.

225. A. False. Water excretion is reduced.
  B. True. Nephrogenic diabetes insipidus.
  C. True. Nephrogenic diabetes insipidus.
  D. True. Cranial diabetes insipidus.
  E. False. Causes inappropriate ADH secretion.
  F. True. Familial condition consisting of diabetes insipidus and one or more of diabetes mellitus, optic atrophy and high-tone deafness.

226. A. True. The increased contribution of glucose to plasma osmolality results in hyponatraemia, without water excess.
  B. True. 'Pseudohyponatraemia' can result if marked hyperlipidaemia contributes significantly to plasma volume, thus reducing the water content per unit volume.
  C. True. Reduced GFR leads to reduced solute delivery to the distal tubules and therefore reduced water excretion.
  D. True. Syndrome of inappropriate ADH secretion.
  E. True. Syndrome of inappropriate ADH secretion.
  F. False. Causes diabetes insipidus; it is of use in the treatment of syndrome of inappropriate ADH secretion.

227. A. False. Inhibits aldosterone effect on distal tubules.
  B. False. May cause hyperkalaemia (angiotensin converting enzyme inhibitor).
  C. True. Increased aldosterone effect.
  D. True. Mineralocorticoid effect.
  E. False. Physiological adrenal replacement maintains normokalaemia.
  F. False. Causes *hyper*kalaemia.

228. A. False. This is true of *extra*cellular pH. Mean intracellular pH is in the range of 6.7–7.3
  B. True. Also bicarbonate/carbonic acid, phosphate and intracellular proteins.
  C. False. This long-term effect occurs over 2–3 days, and is therefore not evident in acute respiratory acidosis.
  D. False. It is a respiratory stimulant, acting on peripheral chemoreceptors.
  E. False. The anion gap is increased by the high plasma levels of negatively charged ketoacids.
  F. True. The anion gap is increased by the high plasma levels of negatively charged lactate.

24. Musculoskeletal and connective tissue disease

229. The following are features of rheumatoid disease:
- **A.** Symmetrical joint involvement.
- **B.** Frequent involvement of the proximal interphalangeal joints.
- **C.** Iritis.
- **D.** Juxta-articular osteoporosis.
- **E.** Trigger finger.
- **F.** Peripheral oedema.

230. In the drug therapy of rheumatoid disease:
- **A.** Non-steroidal anti-inflammatory drugs do not influence the progression of the disease.
- **B.** Gold suppresses disease activity within 2 months.
- **C.** Corticosteroids prevent joint destruction.
- **D.** Intramuscular gold should be continued indefinitely if remission occurs.
- **E.** Daily oral methotrexate is an effective treatment.
- **F.** Sulphasalazine therapy may be complicated by retinal toxicity.

231. In the differential diagnosis of polyarthropathy, the following are true:
- **A.** Reiter's syndrome occurs in young men.
- **B.** Gout occurs commonly in premenopausal women.
- **C.** Systemic lupus erythematosus is more common in women.
- **D.** Rheumatoid disease is more common in men.
- **E.** Association with erythema nodosum suggests chronic sarcoidosis.
- **F.** Pseudogout occurs in the young.

(Answers overleaf)

229. A. **True.**
     B. **True.**
     C. **False.** Episcleritis and scleritis are features of rheumatoid disease.
     D. **True.** Juxta-articular osteoporosis occurs early in the course of rheumatoid disease.
     E. **True.**
     F. **True.** An uncommon manifestation but may affect both the upper and lower limbs.

230. A. **True.** NSAIDs have no disease modifying activity.
     B. **False.** Usually takes at least 3 months.
     C. **False.** No evidence to support this.
     D. **True.** Unless side effects occur.
     E. **False.** Must be given once weekly to minimise toxicity.
     F. **False.** Sulphasalazine causes discolouration of soft contact lenses.

231. A. **True.**
     B. **False.** Gout occurs in postmenopausal women.
     C. **True.** The female: male ratio is 6–9:1.
     D. **False.** Rheumatoid disease is more common in women.
     E. **False.** Acute sarcoidosis is associated with erythema nodosum.
     F. **False.** Occurs in the elderly.

232. The following are features of the anaemia associated with rheumatoid arthritis:
  A. Normal mean cell haemoglobin concentration.
  B. Commonly caused by true iron deficiency.
  C. Inability of the reticuloendothelial cells to release sequestered iron.
  D. Normoblastic bone marrow.
  E. Haemoglobin < 10 g/dl suggests iron deficiency.
  F. Macrocytosis reflects folate status accurately.

233. The seronegative spondarthritides may be differentiated from seropositive rheumatoid disease by:
  A. The presence of HLA-B27.
  B. Atlanto-axial subluxation.
  C. Cartilaginous joint involvement.
  D. Pulmonary effusions.
  E. Symmetrical peripheral joint involvement.
  F. Amyloidosis.

234. In Reiter's syndrome:
  A. *Yersinia enterocolitica* is a recognised cause.
  B. The causative organism can be identified by culture of synovial fluid.
  C. Recurrence of arthritis is typical.
  D. The arthropathy is typically asymmetrical.
  E. Urethritis occurs in the postdysenteric form.
  F. Permanent joint damage is typical.

235. The following are correct statements about osteoarthritis:
  A. The ESR is typically raised.
  B. Heberden's nodes are associated with generalised disease.
  C. The pain is eased by rest.
  D. Morning stiffness is a feature.
  E. Cartilage loss occurs early.
  F. Subchondral cysts occur early in the disease.

(Answers overleaf)

232. A. **False.** The mean cell haemoglobin concentration is typically low.
    B. **False.** It is usually due to chronic disease.
    C. **True.**
    D. **True.** Megaloblastic appearances are rare.
    E. **True.**
    F. **False.** May reflect treatment with azathioprine or methotrexate.

233. A. **True.** HLA-B27 is present in greater than 95% of patients with ankylosing spondylitis.
    B. **False.** Cervical subluxation is a typical feature of seropositive rheumatoid disease.
    C. **True.** The sacro-iliac joints are typically involved in ankylosing spondylitis.
    D. **False.** Apical pulmonary fibrosis occurs in ankylosing spondylitis; pleural effusions in rheumatoid disease.
    E. **True.** Peripheral joint involvement in spondyloarthropathy is usually asymmetrical.
    F. **False.** Amyloidosis may complicate both diseases.

234. A. **True.**
    B. **False.**
    C. **True.** Recurrent attacks occur in more than 60%.
    D. **True.** An asymmetrical arthropathy is typical.
    E. **True.**
    F. **False.** Permanent joint damage is unusual, although arthritis may last for months.

235. A. **False.** Blood tests are normal in uncomplicated osteoarthritis.
    B. **True.**
    C. **True.**
    D. **False.** The pain improves with rest.
    E. **True.**
    F. **False.** A late feature leading to articular surface collapse.

236. The following are true regarding infective arthritis:

A. Tenosynovitis is a feature of gonococcal infection.

B. Gonococcal arthritis occurs more commonly in males.

C. Meningococcal infection characteristically affects large joints.

D. Tuberculous infection presents with an acute monarthritis.

E. Rubella infection resembles acute rheumatoid disease.

F. *Borrelia burgdorferi* causes a recurrent asymmetrical arthritis.

237. In juvenile chronic arthritis (JCA):

A. In systemic JCA the rash is typically purpuric.

B. The arthropathy of systemic JCA is migratory.

C. Rheumatoid factor is typically present.

D. Chronic iridocyclitis is an unusual feature of pauciarticular JCA.

E. The ANA is positive in pauciarticular JCA.

F. There is evidence of preceding streptococcal infection.

238. Gout:

A. Is more common in men.

B. Is rarely caused by thiazide diuretics.

C. Is associated with the presence of negatively birefringent crystals in synovial fluid.

D. Should be treated with allopurinol after the first attack.

E. Is common in chronic renal failure.

F. Joint inflammation results from crystal uptake by polymorphonuclear leucocytes.

239. Features of systemic lupus erythematosus include:

A. A higher incidence in blacks than Caucasians.

B. Raised levels of anti-double-stranded DNA antibodies.

C. Precipitation by hydralazine.

D. Lymphocytosis.

E. Raised serum complement levels which are associated with active disease.

F. Photosensitivity associated with Ro antibodies.

(Answers overleaf)

236. **A. True.**
   B. False. 80% of cases occur in women.
   C. True.
   D. False. Usually presents with a chronic monarthritis.
   E. True.
   F. True. *Borrelia* infection is associated with erythema chronicum migrans.

237. **A. False.** The rash is typically pink, macular and evanescent.
   B. False. This pattern is characteristic of rheumatic fever.
   C. False. Present in < 10% of polyarticular JCA.
   D. False. It is common; children must have a slit lamp examination.
   E. True.
   F. False. This supports the diagnosis of rheumatic fever.

238. **A. True.**
   B. False. Thiazide diuretics are the commonest cause in elderly women.
   C. True. A diagnostic feature.
   D. False. Indications for allopurinol therapy are recurrent attacks, tophi and renal impairment.
   E. False. Hyperuricaemia is common in chronic renal failure but gout is uncommon.
   F. True.

239. **A. True.** The incidence of SLE in black women is 1:250.
   B. True. Anti-double-stranded DNA antibodies are a diagnostic feature.
   C. True.
   D. False. Lymphocytopenia is common.
   E. False. Low C3, C4 and CH50 levels are a feature of active disease.
   F. True.

240. The following are true regarding giant cell arteritis/ polymyalgia rheumatica:

A. Occurs in the elderly.

B. Temporal artery biopsy may be negative in active giant cell arteritis.

C. Blindness occurring in giant cell arteritis is reversible.

D. Histology of affected vessels shows a panarteritis affecting small vessels.

E. The electromyogram is abnormal with polyphasic potentials.

F. The serum creatine phosphokinase is elevated.

241. Features of a prolapsed intervertebral disc:

A. Nerve root compression.

B. A raised ESR.

C. Pain on sneezing.

D. Is common in children.

E. Impairment of urethral sensation.

F. Unremitting night pain.

242. The following are true of soft tissue lesions:

A. Adhesive capsulitis of the shoulder is associated with a normal range of joint movement.

B. In adhesive capsulitis restriction of movement lasts 4–12 weeks.

C. The pain of carpal tunnel syndrome is well localised to the middle and ring fingers.

D. Myxoedema is a cause of carpal tunnel syndrome.

E. Carpal tunnel syndrome usually requires decompression of the ulnar nerve.

F. Fibromyalgia is associated with multiple trigger spots.

(Answers overleaf)

240. **A.** **True.**
    B. **True.** The lesions are not continuous and may be missed on biopsy.
    C. **False.** The blindness is irreversible and may be bilateral.
    D. **False.** Affects large and medium sized vessels.
    E. **False.** The EMG is normal.
    F. **False.** The creatine phosphokinase is normal as are other muscle enzymes.

241. **A.** **True.**
    B. **False.** A raised ESR is a feature of back pain of inflammatory or neoplastic aetiology.
    C. **True.**
    D. **False.** A prolapsed intervertebral disc is uncommon in childhood.
    E. **True.**
    F. **False.**

242. **A.** **False.** Movements of the shoulder are globally reduced in adhesive capsulitis.
    B. **False.** The pain may last 4–12 weeks and the restriction in movement 18 months.
    C. **False.** Pain is frequently poorly localised.
    D. **True.** Also rheumatoid disease, pregnancy, acromegaly and oral contraceptive pill use.
    E. **False.** The median nerve is compressed in the carpal tunnel; may respond to splinting or local cortisone injection.
    F. **True.**

243. The following statements are true:

A. In untreated polymyalgia rheumatica the ESR is usually less than 50 mm/h.

B. α_1-Antitrypsin is an acute-phase protein.

C. Rheumatoid factors are autoantibodies directed against the F(Ab) of IgG.

D. The presence of rheumatoid factors is diagnostic of rheumatoid disease.

E. The lupus anticoagulant is associated with a thrombotic tendency.

F. The C-reactive protein falls more rapidly than the ESR in response to gold therapy.

244. The following are features of dermatomyositis:

A. Symmetrical proximal muscle weakness.

B. Malar erythema.

C. Subcutaneous calcific deposits.

D. Association with malignancy in young patients.

E. Anti-topoisomerase antibodies.

F. Jo-1 antibodies associated with pulmonary disease.

245. The following are true regarding synovial fluid:

A. Normal synovial fluid is a dialysate.

B. Albumin is a major constituent of synovial fluid.

C. Hyaluronic acid is secreted by synovial lining cells.

D. The protein content is increased in synovitis.

E. The viscosity of synovial fluid is increased in inflammatory synovitis.

F. The presence of hyaluronic acid increases the viscosity.

(Answers overleaf)

243. **A.** **False.** In untreated polymyalgia rheumatica the ESR is usually greater than 50 mm/h.
      B. **True.**
      C. **False.** Fc fragments are the targets of rheumatoid factors.
      D. **False.** Rheumatoid factors may be present in other connective tissue and infectious diseases.
      E. **True.**
      F. **True.**

244. **A.** **True.**
      B. **False.** Heliotrope periorbital oedema.
      C. **True.**
      D. **False.** Association with malignancy aged > 50 years.
      E. **False.** Anti-topoisomerase antibodies associated with scleroderma.
      F. **True.**

245. **A.** **True.**
      B. **True.**
      C. **True.**
      D. **True.**
      E. **False.** In inflammatory synovitis the viscosity is decreased.
      F. **True.**

246. Calcium pyrophosphate deposition disease is associated with:

A. Hypocalcaemia.
B. Hyperthyroidism.
C. Weakly positive birefrigent crystals in synovial fluid.
D. Chondrocalcinosis of the triangular ligament of the wrist.
E. Haemochromatosis.
F. Wilson's disease.

247. Features of polyarteritis nodosa include:

A. Multiple aneurysm formation.
B. Upper respiratory tract involvement.
C. Association with hepatitis A infection.
D. Panarteritis.
E. Livedo reticularis.
F. Eosinophilia.

248. The following are features of Behçet's disease:

A. Aphthous oral ulceration.
B. Scleritis.
C. Meningoencephalitis.
D. Chronic arthropathy of weight-bearing joints.
E. Eye disease which responds well to cyclosporin A.
F. Erythema marginatum.

(Answers overleaf)

246. **A.** **False.** Hypercalcaemia is associated with this disease.
    B. **False.** Hypothyroidism is associated with this disease.
    C. **True.**
    D. **True.** A typical site for chondrocalcinosis, other sites are the knee menisci and the pubic symphysis.
    E. **True.**
    F. **True.**

247. **A.** **True.**
    B. **False.** Suggests Wegener's granulomatosis.
    C. **False.** Hepatitis B infection is associated with polyarteritis nodosa.
    D. **True.**
    E. **True.**
    F. **False.** Suggests Churg–Strauss syndrome.

248. **A.** **True.**
    B. **False.** Iritis is a feature of Behçet's disease.
    C. **True.**
    D. **True.**
    E. **True.**
    F. **False.** Erythema nodosum occurs in Behçet's disease.

25. Haematological disorders

249. The oxygen affinity of haemoglobin:
A. Is reduced by a rise in temperature.
B. Is increased by a fall in pH.
C. Is reduced by a rise in 2,3-diphosphoglycerate level.
D. Is reduced in chronic anaemia.
E. Is independent of the Po_2.
F. Is raised in polycythaemia rubra vera.

250. The following suggest a diagnosis of iron deficiency anaemia:
A. Koilonychia.
B. Low total iron binding capacity.
C. Anisocytosis on blood film.
D. Low serum ferritin.
E. Pencil cells on blood film.
F. Decreased cellular expression of the transferrin receptor.

251. Vitamin B_{12} deficiency may result from:
A. Gastrectomy.
B. Crohn's disease.
C. Phenytoin treatment.
D. Myxoedema.
E. Pancreatic insufficiency.
F. Potassium supplements.

252. In hypoplastic anaemia:
A. The reticulocyte count is usually raised.
B. The disease may result from therapy with thiouracil drugs.
C. Splenomegaly is found in most cases.
D. The platelet count is usually normal.
E. The disease may respond to immunosuppressive therapy.
F. The risk of rejection of a bone marrow transplant is reduced by the removal of mature T cells from the marrow inoculum.

(Answers overleaf)

249. A. **True.**
   B. **False.** It is reduced by a fall in pH; this leads to increased tissue oxygen delivery.
   C. **True.** This stabilises the deoxygenated form.
   D. **True.** This is due to a rise in 2,3-DPG levels.
   E. **False.** The binding of oxygen to haem increases the oxygen affinity.
   F. **False.** It is normal; high-affinity haemoglobin is a cause of secondary polycythaemia.

250. A. **True.**
   B. **False.** Serum iron is low, total iron binding capacity is high/normal.
   C. **True.** Also poikilocytosis.
   D. **True.**
   E. **True.** Narrow elliptocytes.
   F. **False.** Expression of the transferrin receptor is increased; this is mediated by upregulation of the iron-responsive element-binding protein (IRE-BP).

251. A. **True.** Lack of intrinsic factor.
   B. **True.** Terminal ileal disease.
   C. **False.** This treatment causes folate deficiency.
   D. **False.** However, it can cause a macrocytic anaemia.
   E. **True.** This causes B_{12} malabsorption by reducing terminal ileal pH and Ca^{2+} concentration.
   F. **True.** These inhibit B_{12} absorption.

252. A. **False.** The reticulocyte count is low.
   B. **True.** An idiosyncratic reaction.
   C. **False.** Splenomegaly would suggest another cause for the pancytopenia.
   D. **False.** It is reduced in most cases.
   E. **True.** High-dose steroids, cyclosporin or anti-lymphocyte serum.
   F. **False.** This reduces graft-versus-host disease, but increases the risk of rejection.

253. The following are true of congenital haemolytic anaemias:

A. A microcytic anaemia is consistent with a diagnosis of thalassaemia.
B. Hypersplenism is common in sickle cell disease.
C. Hereditary elliptocytosis is an X-linked recessive condition.
D. Sulphonamides may precipitate haemolysis in glucose-6-phosphate dehydrogenase deficiency.
E. Aplastic crises in sickle cell disease may be precipitated by Coxsackie virus infections.
F. Levels of HbF are raised in β-thalassaemia major.

254. Causes of autoimmune haemolytic anaemia include:

A. Chronic lymphocytic leukaemia.
B. Infectious mononucleosis.
C. Cardiac valve replacement.
D. Systemic lupus erythematosus.
E. Cobra venom.
F. Haemolytic uraemic syndrome.

255. In a patient with blood group A Rh-negative:

A. The serum will contain anti-B IgM antibodies.
B. The red cells will agglutinate with anti-A+B serum.
C. The serum will contain agglutinating anti-D antibodies.
D. The serum will agglutinate group O red cells.
E. The red cells will agglutinate with anti-D serum in an indirect antiglobulin test.
F. The rhesus genotype may be CDe/cde.

256. In immune haemolytic disease of the newborn:

A. Fetal haemolysis is caused by maternal IgM antibodies crossing the placenta.
B. The disease is usually most severe in the first-born child.
C. Nucleated red cells are found in the fetal peripheral blood.
D. The mother may have blood group O Rh-positive.
E. Severe hyperbilirubinaemia occurs *in utero*.
F. Falling levels of maternal anti-D antibody during the third trimester indicate an affected fetus.

(Answers overleaf)

253. A. **True.**
    B. **False.** Splenic infarcts lead to hyposplenism.
    C. **False.** It is an autosomal dominant condition.
    D. **True.** Many drugs are implicated.
    E. **False.** Usually by parvovirus infections.
    F. **True.** Production of α- and γ-chains is normal or increased.

254. A. **True.** It can occur secondary to any malignancy.
    B. **True.** Cold antibodies with *i* blood group specificity.
    C. **False.** Haemolysis is due to red cell trauma.
    D. **True.** It can occur in all autoimmune diseases.
    E. **False.** Haemolysis is due to a non-immune toxic effect.
    F. **False.** Microangiopathic haemolytic anaemia.

255. A. **True.** Complete antibodies; they will agglutinate red cells in the cold.
    B. **True.** They agglutinate also with anti-A, but not with anti-B serum.
    C. **False.** Anti-D antibodies do not occur naturally and are IgG, non-agglutinating.
    D. **False.** Group O cells do not react with either anti-A or anti-B sera.
    E. **False.** However, Rh-positive red cells will.
    F. **False.** It must be d/d.

256. A. **False.** IgG.
    B. **False.** Maternal sensitisation usually occurs in the first pregnancy, and only subsequent pregnancies are affected.
    C. **True.** Erythroblastosis fetalis.
    D. **True.** It may rarely be due to incompatibility of non-rhesus blood group systems including ABO.
    E. **False.** Not until after birth, as bilirubin is cleared by the placenta.
    F. **False.** Rising levels of anti-D.

257. The following are recognised causes of lymphopenia:

A. Megaloblastic anaemia.
B. Lymphoma.
C. Typhoid.
D. Pertussis.
E. Exposure to irradiation.
F. Kostman's syndrome.

258. In chronic myeloid leukaemia:

A. Lymphadenopathy is common.
B. Most patients are over 30 years of age.
C. The neutrophil alkaline phosphatase level is usually very low.
D. Recurrent infections are a common presenting feature.
E. The peripheral blood basophil count is often elevated.
F. Lymphoblasts may be seen in the peripheral blood in acute transformation.

259. In polycythaemia rubra vera:

A. Erythropoietin production is increased.
B. Plasma volume is normal or increased.
C. Oxygen saturation is normal.
D. The platelet count may be raised.
E. Peptic ulceration is due to increased gastrin secretion.
F. Serum B_{12} level is reduced.

260. The following are true of acute lymphoblastic leukaemia:

A. The incidence peaks between the ages of 10 and 15.
B. Central nervous system involvement is common at presentation.
C. The anaemia is usually normocytic.
D. The prognosis is worse in males.
E. Auer rods may be seen in the lymphoblasts.
F. The Philadelphia chromosome may be present.

(Answers overleaf)

257. **A.** **True.** If severe.
   B. **True.**
   C. **False.** It may cause neutropenia.
   D. **False.** Lymphocytosis is common.
   E. **True.**
   F. **False.** This is a form of congenital neutropenia.

258. **A.** **False.** It is rare, but splenomegaly is almost invariable.
   B. **True.** However, childhood variants occur.
   C. **True.** It is high in other myeloproliferative disorders and reactive leucocytosis.
   D. **False.** They are rare at presentation.
   E. **True.** There is an increase in neutrophils, eosinophils and basophils.
   F. **True.** They are seen in about 20% of blast crises; myeloblasts are seen in the other 80%.

259. **A.** **False.** This occurs in secondary polycythaemia.
   B. **True.** Plasma volume is reduced in pseudopolycythaemia.
   C. **True.** Reduced oxygen saturation leads to secondary polycythaemia.
   D. **True.** This occurs in about 50% of patients.
   E. **False.** It is due to hyperviscosity and increased histamine release from basophils.
   F. **False.** B_{12} level is raised secondary to increased B_{12} binding protein release.

260. **A.** **False.** The incidence peaks at the age of 5 then falls in adolescence.
   B. **False.** It is rare at presentation, but is a common site of relapse without craniospinal prophylaxis.
   C. **True.**
   D. **True.**
   E. **False.** They are seen in myeloblasts in acute myeloid leukaemia.
   F. **True.** This is so in 5% of childhood and 20% of adult cases.

261. In Hodgkin's disease:
A. Spread is predominantly via the lymphatics in the early stages.
B. The lymphocyte-predominant histological type has a poor prognosis.
C. Nodal involvement on both sides of the diaphragm is classified as stage II in the Ann Arbor system.
D. The presence of systemic symptoms does not affect the overall prognosis.
E. Eosinophilia occurs in up to 15% of cases.
F. Patients with stage IIIB disease may be treated with radiotherapy alone.

262. The following are true of chronic lymphocytic leukaemia:
A. It occurs predominantly in the elderly.
B. It is more common in males than females.
C. Lymphadenopathy is unusual at presentation.
D. The median survival is about 6 months.
E. The proliferating lymphocytes are B cells in most cases.
F. Steroid treatment is contraindicated.

263. The following are recognised features of multiple myeloma:
A. Osteoporotic bone lesions.
B. Overall median survival of 2–3 years.
C. Free immunoglobulin heavy chains in the urine.
D. Impaired humoral immunity.
E. Peripheral neuropathy.
F. Reduced serum β_2 microglobulin level.

264. The following features support a diagnosis of amyloidosis:
A. Peripheral neuropathy.
B. Macroglossia.
C. Dilated cardiomyopathy.
D. Arthropathy.
E. Acute nephritic syndrome.
F. Signs of chronic liver disease.

(Answers overleaf)

261. **A.** **True.** Involved nodes are commonly contiguous.
     B. **False.** It has a good prognosis.
     C. **False.** It is classified as stage III.
     D. **False.** The prognosis is worse.
     E. **True.**
     F. **False.** Chemotherapy is essential for stages IIIB and IV.

262. **A.** **True.** The incidence rises steeply with advanced age.
     B. **True.** It is almost twice as common in males.
     C. **False.** Most cases present with it.
     D. **False.** It exceeds 5 years.
     E. **True.** In over 95% of cases.
     F. **False.** It may be of value if there is associated thrombocytopenia or autoimmune haemolytic anaemia.

263. **A.** **True.** The proliferating plasma cells release an osteoclast activating factor.
     B. **True.**
     C. **False.** Free light chains (Bence-Jones' proteinuria).
     D. **True.** Normal antibody production is suppressed.
     E. **True.** A non-metastatic effect.
     F. **False.** The level is usually raised and is a useful prognostic indicator.

264. **A.** **True.**
     B. **True.**
     C. **False.** Restrictive cardiomyopathy.
     D. **True.**
     E. **False.** Renal involvement commonly causes nephrotic syndrome.
     F. **False.** Liver infiltration is common, but liver function is not impaired.

265. In the coagulation cascade:
  A. Factor IXa converts prothrombin to thrombin.
  B. Factor VII is activated by tissue thromboplastins in the extrinsic cascade.
  C. The activation of factor X requires magnesium ions.
  D. Factor XIII catalyses fibrin cross-linkage.
  E. Antithrombin III activates the fibrinolytic system.
  F. Protein C inactivates factors V and VIII.

266. The following are causes of a prolonged prothrombin time:
  A. Liver disease.
  B. Warfarin treatment.
  C. Heparin treatment.
  D. Haemophilia A.
  E. Von Willebrand's disease.
  F. Factor VII deficiency.

267. The following are recognised causes of thrombocytosis:
  A. Postsplenectomy.
  B. Sarcoidosis.
  C. Haemolytic uraemic syndrome.
  D. Myeloproliferative disease.
  E. Wiskott–Aldrich syndrome.
  F. Thiazide diuretics.

268. In haemophilia A:
  A. The diagnosis may be made antenatally.
  B. The inheritance is autosomal recessive.
  C. The thrombin time is normal.
  D. The disease is mild if the level of factor VIIIC is over 5% of normal.
  E. Recombinant factor VIII should no longer be used because of the risk of viral transmission.
  F. The half-life of injected factor VIII is in the order of 48 hours.

(Answers overleaf)

265. A. False. Factor Xa converts prothrombin.
   B. True.
   C. False. It requires calcium ions.
   D. True.
   E. False. It inhibits thrombin and factors IXa, Xa and XIa.
   F. True.

266. A. True. This causes reduced production of vitamin-K-dependent factors and factor V.
   B. True. It interferes with the production of vitamin-K-dependent factors.
   C. True. It increases the activity of antithrombin III.
   D. False. Factor VIII is involved only in the intrinsic pathway.
   E. False. The PT is normal, but the bleeding time and, usually, the APTT are prolonged.
   F. True. Factor VII is part of the extrinsic pathway.

267. A. True. Usually transient.
   B. True. It can occur in any inflammatory condition.
   C. False. Thrombocytopenia due to microangiopathic platelet destruction.
   D. True. Primary thrombocytosis.
   E. False. Hereditary immunodeficiency and thrombocytopenia.
   F. False. These are a rare cause of reduced platelet production.

268. A. True. The diagnosis is made either by measurement of the factor VIIIC level in fetal blood or by analysis of chorionic villus DNA.
   B. False. It is X-linked recessive.
   C. True. The test bypasses the intrinsic (and extrinsic) pathway.
   D. True.
   E. False. It carries no risk, unlike some factor VIII concentrates.
   F. False. The half-life is 12 hours; it has to be administered twice daily during a severe bleeding episode.

26. Neurological disease

269. The following are true regarding visual field defects:

A. A midline lesion of the optic chiasm causes a bitemporal hemianopia.

B. A lesion of the optic tract causes a homonymous hemianopia.

C. A suprasellar meningioma causes an upper bitemporal hemianopia.

D. An expanding pituitary tumour causes a lower bitemporal hemianopia.

E. A lesion of the lower and lateral part of the optic radiation in the parietal lobe causes an upper quadrantanopia.

F. A complete lesion of both occipital lobes causes cortical blindness with loss of the pupillary reflexes.

270. Causes of papilloedema include:

A. Optic neuritis.

B. Multiple sclerosis.

C. Central retinal vein occlusion.

D. Hypertension.

E. Pituitary tumour.

F. Retinitis pigmentosa.

271. The following are true statements:

A. The IIIrd cranial nerve supplies the superior oblique muscle.

B. A VIth cranial nerve palsy produces impairment of abduction of the eye.

C. A complete IIIrd cranial nerve lesion results in an impaired or absent pupillary reflex.

D. The Holmes–Adie pupil is constricted and irregular.

E. Horner's syndrome is caused by lesions of the cervical parasympathetic supply.

F. A lower motor neurone lesion of the VIIth cranial nerve will affect all the muscles of facial expression.

(Answers overleaf)

269. **A. True.**
   B. True.
   C. False. Pressure on the optic chiasm from above, usually due to a suprasellar meningioma, produces a lower bitemporal quadrantanopia.
   D. False. An expanding pituitary tumour from below will produce an upper bitemporal quadrantanopia, due to the inversion of the image on the retina.
   E. True.
   F. False. The pupillary reflexes are preserved.

270. **A. True.**
   B. True.
   C. True.
   D. True.
   E. False.
   F. False.

271. **A. False.** The IIIrd nerve supplies the extraocular muscles except the lateral rectus (VIth nerve) and superior oblique (IVth nerve) muscles.
   B. True.
   C. True. The pupil is typically dilated and fixed to light.
   D. False. The Holmes–Adie pupil is large with a poor response to light.
   E. False. Horner's syndrome is due to lesions of the cervical sympathetic supply.
   F. True. An upper motor neurone VIIth nerve lesion only affects the lower half of the face because the frontal muscles are bilaterally innervated.

272. Features of migraine include:

A. Pain which is worse in the evening.
B. Preceding visual symptoms.
C. An elevated ESR.
D. Normal neurological examination following an attack.
E. Continuous pain lasting 7 days.
F. Night-time waking.

273. The following are true regarding epilepsy:

A. Simple partial seizures are followed by loss of consciousness.
B. Petit mal attacks last for several minutes.
C. Treatment should not be started after the first fit.
D. Patients who have two or more daytime fits may not drive for one year.
E. Carbamazepine does not impair the efficacy of the oral contraceptive pill.
F. Three-second spike-and-wave discharges on the electroencephalogram are diagnostic of petit mal epilepsy.

274. Transient ischaemic attacks:

A. Resolve completely within 24 hours.
B. Should be treated with low-dose aspirin to reduce the risk of further stroke.
C. Are typically caused by cardiac emboli.
D. Should usually be treated by anticoagulation.
E. May lead to amaurosis fugax caused by posterior cerebral artery embolism.
F. In the vertebrobasilar territory can cause a hemiparesis.

275. In stroke:

A. The onset is typically abrupt.
B. A middle cerebral artery occlusion affects the contralateral leg more severely than the arm.
C. An ipsilateral Horner's syndrome is a feature of posterior inferior cerebellar artery occlusion.
D. Intracerebral haemorrhage is more common than cerebral infarction.
E. Intracranial haemorrhage is often clinically indistinguishable from intracranial infarction.
F. Cerebral oedema is maximal 4–7 days after cerebral infarction.

(Answers overleaf)

272. **A.** **False.** Typical of tension headache.
   B. **True.** Visual symptoms are a feature of migraine.
   C. **False.** A raised ESR is a feature of giant cell arteritis, which requires further investigation and urgent treatment with prednisolone to prevent blindness.
   D. **True.** An abnormal neurological examination suggests intracranial pathology.
   E. **False.** A typical feature of tension headaches.
   F. **False.** Migraine headaches rarely waken the patient at night.

273. **A.** **False.** Complex partial seizures are followed by loss of consciousness.
   B. **False.** Petit mal type absence attacks last 10–15 seconds.
   C. **False.** The risk of further fits in the next 2 years is 70%, but most patients opt not to start treatment after a single fit.
   D. **False.** Patients are banned from driving until fit free for at least one year.
   E. **False.** Carbamazepine induces liver enzymes and hence increases the metabolism of oestrogens and reduces the efficacy of the oral contraceptive pill.
   F. **True.**

274. **A.** **True.** This is the definition of a transient ischaemic attack.
   B. **True.**
   C. **False.** Only 5–10% of patients with transient ischaemic attacks have a demonstrable source of cardiac emboli.
   D. **False.** Anticoagulation should only be started if a continuing source of cardiac emboli is present.
   E. **False.** Amaurosis fugax is usually caused by retinal emboli (carotid territory).
   F. **True.**

275. **A.** **True.** A cardinal feature.
   B. **False.** The arm is more affected than the leg in a middle cerebral artery occlusion, because the leg area of the cortex is relatively spared.
   C. **True.** Caused by involvement of the descending sympathetic fibres in the reticular formation.
   D. **False.** Cerebral infarction causes eight times as many strokes as cerebral haemorrhage.
   E. **True.** The distinction can be made by computerised tomography.
   F. **True.** Cerebral oedema after infarction resolves over 2–4 weeks.

276. The following are true of subarachnoid haemorrhage:
   A. The headache is of sudden onset.
   B. A third nerve palsy can occur as a result of an expanding posterior communicating artery aneurysm.
   C. Subhyaloid haemorrhages are a feature.
   D. Subarachnoid haemorrhage is associated with adult polycystic kidney disease.
   E. Xanthochromia develops in the cerebrospinal fluid within the first 24 hours.
   F. The risk of rebleeding is maximal in the first 7 days.

277. Alzheimer's disease:
   A. May be mimicked by depression.
   B. Is an unusual cause of dementia in the elderly.
   C. Causes focal atrophy of the frontal and temporal lobes.
   D. Causes antisocial behaviour as a late feature.
   E. Has as a pathological feature neurofibrillary tangles.
   F. Is associated with abnormal apolipoprotein E4 genotype.

278. The following are true of cerebral tumours:
   A. Grade I astrocytomas have a poor prognosis.
   B. Meningiomas arise from the arachnoid.
   C. Meningiomas are rapidly growing malignant tumours.
   D. Cerebellopontine angle tumours present with ipsilateral progressive deafness.
   E. Medulloblastomas commonly occur in adults.
   F. Medulloblastomas arise in the roof of the fourth ventricle.

279. In the drug treatment of Parkinson's disease:
   A. Levodopa has the greatest effect on tremor.
   B. Levodopa should be given with an extracerebral decarboxylase inhibitor.
   C. Side-effects of levodopa include agitation.
   D. Anticholinergic drugs are contraindicated in glaucoma.
   E. Akinesia should be treated with anticholinergic drugs.
   F. Selegiline increases levels of dopamine.

(Answers overleaf)

276. **A.** **True.**
     B. **True.**
     C. **True.**   Subhyaloid haemorrhages are only seen in subarachnoid haemorrhage.
     D. **True.**   10–20% of patients with adult polycystic kidney disease have intracranial aneurysms.
     E. **False.**   Xanthochromia does not develop for at least 24 hours.
     F. **False.**   The risk of rebleed is maximal at 7–14 days.

277. **A.** **True.**   Depression is the commonest cause of pseudodementia.
     B. **False.**   Commonest cause of dementia in people aged over 60 years.
     C. **False.**   Frontal lobe atrophy is a typical feature of Pick's disease.
     D. **False.**   A common early feature of Alzheimer's disease.
     E. **True.**
     F. **True.**   In some familial cases.

278. **A.** **False.**   Grade I astrocytomas have the best prognosis and grade IV the worst with a < 20% 1-year survival.
     B. **True.**
     C. **False.**   Meningiomas are benign and usually slow-growing tumours.
     D. **True.**   However, in cases due to a meningioma there may not be deafness.
     E. **False.**   Medulloblastomas nearly always occur in children.
     F. **True.**

279. **A.** **False.**   The main effect of levodopa is on akinesia.
     B. **True.**   Reduces peripheral breakdown of levodopa, permitting use of lower doses with less side-effects.
     C. **True.**
     D. **True.**   Anticholinergic drugs may precipitate acute glaucoma.
     E. **False.**   The major effect of anticholinergic drugs is on tremor.
     F. **True.**

280. The following statements about tremor are correct:

A. A rest tremor is typical of Parkinson's disease.
B. The tremor of Parkinson's disease is exacerbated by movement.
C. An action tremor is likely to be due to a cerebellar cause.
D. Asterixis occurs in renal failure.
E. Postural tremor is a feature of hypothyroidism.
F. Multiple sclerosis is a cause of an action tremor.

281. The following statements are true about spinal cord lesions:

A. A unilateral lesion of the corticospinal tracts below the level of the lower medulla will cause an ipsilateral motor weakness.
B. A lesion of the dorsal columns will affect pain and temperature sensation.
C. An acute spinal cord transection gives rise to a spastic paraparesis.
D. In the Brown-Séquard syndrome there is ipsilateral loss of pain and temperature sensation.
E. A lesion at C3 or above may cause respiratory paralysis.
F. A sensory level gives an accurate indication of the level of a spinal lesion.

282. The following are features of cervical spondylosis:

A. The commonest level is at C1/2.
B. Cord compression may develop acutely.
C. Pain and parasthesiae occur in a root distribution.
D. The upper limb reflexes are all depressed with a C5/6 lesion.
E. An inverted supinator jerk describes a finger jerk occurring when the biceps reflex is elicited.
F. Presents with a dissociated sensory loss.

283. Features of motor neurone disease include:

A. Anterior horn cell involvement.
B. Involvement of the motor neurones to the bladder.
C. Fasciculation.
D. Sensory loss.
E. Electromyography shows denervation of clinically uninvolved muscle groups.
F. A slowly progressive course.

(Answers overleaf)

280. **A. True.**
 B. False. The tremor of Parkinson's disease is improved by movement.
 C. True.
 D. True.
 E. False. Postural tremor is a feature of hyperthyroidism.
 F. True.

281. **A. True.** The corticospinal tracts decussate at the level of the lower medulla.
 B. False. The dorsal columns carry joint position sense, vibration and some touch sensation.
 C. False. Acute spinal cord lesions result in a flaccid paraplegia with areflexia and non-reactive plantar responses.
 D. False. Pain and temperature loss is contralateral to the lesion in the Brown-Séquard syndrome.
 E. True. Lesions at or above C3 affect the phrenic nerve and cause respiratory paralysis.
 F. False. A sensory level localizes the lesion to the spinal cord, but the lesion may be several segments above the sensory level.

282. **A. False.** C5/6 is the commonest level.
 B. True. As a result of a central disc prolapse.
 C. True.
 D. False. The biceps and supinator jerks are depressed, but other reflexes are brisk.
 E. True.
 F. False. A feature of a cervical syrinx or other intrinsic cord lesion.

283. **A. True.**
 B. False. The motor neurones to the bladder are typically spared.
 C. True.
 D. False. Sensation is not affected.
 E. True.
 F. False. The course is rapid, death usually occurring within 3–4 years of onset of symptoms.

284. Features of median nerve entrapment at the wrist include:
   A. Pain in the hand worst at night.
   B. Weakness of adductor pollicis brevis.
   C. Sensory loss over the palmar surface of the ring and middle fingers.
   D. A positive Finkelstein's test.
   E. Weakness of the long flexors of the fingers.
   F. Weakness of the medial two lumbrical muscles.

285. Features of the Guillain–Barré syndrome include:
   A. Respiratory muscle weakness.
   B. Involvement of the autonomic nervous system.
   C. Proximal paraesthesiae among the first symptoms.
   D. Weakness is usually maximal 10–14 days after onset of neuropathy.
   E. Normal CSF protein.
   F. Bladder dysfunction.

286. Recognized features of Duchenne muscular dystrophy include:
   A. Onset of symptoms between 5 and 25 years of age.
   B. Location of the abnormal gene on the short arm of the X chromosome.
   C. Cardiac failure.
   D. Wasting of calf muscles.
   E. Normal creatine kinase at birth.
   F. Painful muscles.

287. In myasthenia gravis:
   A. Anti-acetylcholine receptor antibody titres are raised.
   B. Thymoma is associated in older patients.
   C. Fatigable weakness of smooth muscle is characteristic.
   D. The titre of anti-acetylcholine receptor antibodies is a useful guide to severity.
   E. Treatment is with the long-acting cholinesterase pyridostigmine.
   F. Neonatal myasthenia gravis occurs as a result of placental transfer of IgM anti-acetylcholine receptor antibodies.

(Answers overleaf)

284. **A.** **True.**
    B. **False.** Abductor pollicis brevis is affected.
    C. **True.**
    D. **False.** Tinel's sign (tapping over the carpal tunnel producing paraesthesiae) and Phalen's sign (wrist flexion reproducing the symptoms) may be positive. Finkelstein's sign is present in de Quervain's tenosynovitis.
    E. **False.** A feature of median nerve lesion at the elbow.
    F. **False.** The medial two lumbrical muscles are supplied by the ulnar nerve.

285. **A.** **True.** Respiratory muscle weakness may be severe enough to need ventilatory support.
    B. **True.** Autonomic involvement can cause lability of blood pressure.
    C. **False.** Distal paraesthesiae are among the first symptoms.
    D. **True.**
    E. **False.** The CSF protein is elevated to 1–10 g/l.
    F. **False.** Bladder dysfunction is rare.

286. **A.** **False.** Most affected boys are in a wheelchair by age 10 and dead by age 20. The Becker type presents between the ages of 5 and 25 years.
    B. **True.** The mutation is in the gene for dystrophin, which is located on the short arm of the X chromosome.
    C. **True.** Cardiac failure is a common cause of death.
    D. **False.** The calf muscles show pseudohypertrophy together with the deltoids.
    E. **False.** The creatine kinase is elevated at birth.
    F. **False.** The weakness is painless.

287. **A.** **True.** Anti-acetylcholine receptor antibodies are raised in 90% of patients.
    B. **True.**
    C. **False.** Striated muscle is affected.
    D. **False.** There is a poor correlation between the titre of anti-acetylcholine receptor antibodies and severity of disease.
    E. **False.** Pyridostigmine is a cholinesterase inhibitor.
    F. **False.** IgG anti-acetylcholine receptor antibodies cross the placenta.

288. Features of diabetic neuropathy include:

A. Involvement of the IIIrd cranial nerve.

B. Painless amyotrophy.

C. Sensorimotor involvement commonly.

D. Postural hypotension.

E. Distal amyotrophy.

F. Microangiopathy.

289. In multiple sclerosis:

A. There is an increased prevalence in tropical climates.

B. Corticosteroids may accelerate recovery from acute relapse.

C. Demyelination of peripheral nerves occurs.

D. Optic neuritis with a central scotoma is a common initial feature.

E. MRI is the investigation of choice.

F. A relapsing remitting course is more likely to occur at younger age of onset.

290. The following statements about bacterial meningitis are correct:

A. *Neisseria meningitidis* infection should be treated with intrathecal benzyl penicillin.

B. A purpuric rash is a typical feature of *Streptococcus pneumoniae* meningitis.

C. The CSF typically shows a glucose level greater than 40% of the blood glucose.

D. Fits are a common presenting feature in the young.

E. Rifampicin should be used to treat close contacts of patients with *Neisseria meningitidis*.

F. VIIIth nerve damage is usually transient.

291. Recognized features of tuberculous meningitis include:

A. Infection with atypical mycobacteria in many cases.

B. An acute presentation in most cases.

C. Cranial nerve palsies.

D. Inappropriate antidiuretic hormone secretion.

E. Low CSF glucose.

F. A requirement for therapy with four antituberculous drugs.

(Answers overleaf)

288. A. True.
    B. False. Amyotrophy is painful.
    C. True.
    D. True. Usually associated with a sensorimotor neuropathy.
    E. False. Amyotrophy occurs proximally.
    F. True.

289. A. False. Is a disease of temperate climates.
    B. True.
    C. False. Peripheral nerves are not affected by demyelination.
    D. True.
    E. True.
    F. True.

290. A. False. Intrathecal antibiotics are hazardous and do not improve the outcome.
    B. False. A typical feature of *Neisseria meningitidis* infection.
    C. False. The CSF glucose is < 40% of the blood glucose.
    D. True. Fits are not a common presenting feature in adults.
    E. True.
    F. False. Deafness may be bilateral, severe and permanent.

291. A. False. Atypical mycobacteria are unusual causes of tuberculous meningitis.
    B. False. Usually presents subacutely.
    C. True.
    D. True.
    E. True.
    F. True.

292. Neurological features of the acquired immunodeficiency syndrome include:

A. *Toxoplasma gondii* cerebral abscess.

B. Direct infection of nerve cells by the human immunodeficiency virus.

C. CMV retinitis.

D. *Cryptococcus neoformans* meningitis.

E. Myopathy associated with zidovudine therapy.

F. Symmetrical painless sensory motor neuropathy.

293. The effects of alcohol on the nervous system include:

A. Auditory hallucinations which are a typical feature of delirium tremens.

B. A progressive dementia which improves with total abstinence from alcohol.

C. A normal electroencephalogram following alcohol withdrawal fits.

D. A painful peripheral neuropathy.

E. An acute direct inhibitory effect on neuronal cell membranes.

F. Alcohol withdrawal fits which typically occur within 12 hours.

294. Cavernous sinus thrombosis:

A. Occurs secondary to facial infection.

B. Is characterised by pulsatile proptosis.

C. Should be treated with high-dose intravenous antibiotics.

D. Is characterised by pain in the affected eye.

E. Is associated with facial sensory impairment secondary to trigeminal nerve involvement.

F. Is associated with loss of visual acuity in the affected eye.

295. Features of the Wernicke–Korsakoff syndrome:

A. Occurrence solely in alcoholics.

B. Peripheral neuropathy.

C. A confabulatory dementia which responds well to treatment with thiamine.

D. Thiamine deficiency.

E. Nystagmus.

F. Elevation of the red cell transketolase.

(Answers overleaf)

292. **A.** **True.** *Toxoplasma gondii* cerebral abscesses occur in 70% of patients.
  B. **True.** The human immunodeficiency virus is highly neurotropic.
  C. **True.**
  D. **True.**
  E. **True.**
  F. **False.** The peripheral neuropathy is painful.

293. **A.** **False.** Visual hallucinations are a more typical feature.
  B. **True.** In the early stages abstinence from alcohol may improve the dementia.
  C. **True.**
  D. **True.** Pain is characteristic of alcoholic peripheral neuropathy.
  E. **True.**
  F. **False.** Alcohol withdrawal fits occur within 12–48 hours after alcohol withdrawal.

294. **A.** **True.**
  B. **False.** A feature of caroticocavernous fistula.
  C. **True.**
  D. **True.**
  E. **True.**
  F. **True.**

295. **A.** **False.** Occurs in other states of thiamine deficiency.
  B. **True.** A peripheral neuropathy is present in 80% of patients.
  C. **False.** The confabulatory dementia responds poorly to thiamine treatment.
  D. **True.**
  E. **True.**
  F. **False.** The red cell transketolase is reduced.

296. In the examination of the CSF:

A. Lumbar puncture may be safely performed in the presence of coma.

B. In tuberculous meningitis more than 1000 cells/mm³ are present.

C. In viral meningitis the glucose is commonly low.

D. The protein is raised in tuberculous meningitis.

E. The glucose may be low in subarachnoid haemorrhage.

F. *Cryptococcus neoformans* may be demonstrated by Indian ink staining.

297. Features of dystrophia myotonica (myotonic dystrophy) include:

A. Genetic anticipation.

B. Proximal myotonia as an early feature.

C. Normal intelligence.

D. Normal reproductive capacity.

E. Presentation in the age range 20–40 years.

F. Frontal balding in females.

298. Subacute combined degeneration of the cord:

A. Is due to deficiency of vitamin B_2.

B. Is due to degeneration of the spinothalamic tracts.

C. Features optic atrophy.

D. Is excluded by the presence of a normal haemoglobin.

E. Is characterised by a raised mean corpuscular volume.

F. Is treated with oral vitamin B_{12}.

(Answers overleaf)

296. **A. False.** There is a risk of coning. Computerised tomography should be performed first.
   B. False. In tuberculous meningitis the CSF contains 50–500 cells/mm^3.
   C. False. In viral meningitis the blood sugar is rarely low, this suggests bacterial infection.
   D. True. A differentiating feature from viral infection.
   E. True.
   F. True. Indian ink staining is a useful method of detecting fungal infection of the CSF.

297. **A. True.** The gene is on chromosone 19.
   B. False. Proximal muscle myotonia is a late feature.
   C. False. The intelligence is low.
   D. False. There is gonadal atrophy.
   E. True.
   F. False. A feature in males.

298. **A. False.** There is a deficiency of vitamin B$_{12}$.
   B. False. The lateral and posterior columns degenerate, together with a peripheral neuropathy.
   C. True.
   D. False. The haemoglobin may be normal.
   E. True. The mean corpuscular volume is invariably raised.
   F. False. Treatment is with parenteral vitamin B$_{12}$.

299. Features of Friedreich's ataxia include:
   A. Autosomal recessive inheritance.
   B. Ataxia of gait and limbs which develops in adulthood.
   C. Axonal sensory neuropathy with areflexia.
   D. Cutaneous telangiectasia.
   E. Diabetes mellitus.
   F. Cardiomyopathy.

300. Creutzfeldt–Jakob disease:
   A. Has a viral aetiology.
   B. Causes a spongiform encephalopathy.
   C. Is characterised by ataxia as a feature.
   D. Is slowly progressive.
   E. May be transmitted by corneal grafts.
   F. Shows pathological similarities to kuru.

(Answers overleaf)

299. A. **True.**
     B. **False.** Onset is usually in childhood. Always before the age of 25 years.
     C. **True.**
     D. **False.** A feature of ataxia telangiectasia.
     E. **True.** Diabetes mellitus is present in 10% of patients.
     F. **True.** Cardiomyopathy is present in 66% of patients.

300. A. **False.** Is due to infectious prion proteins.
     B. **True.**
     C. **True.**
     D. **False.** 70% mortality at 6 months.
     E. **True.**
     F. **True.**